Glossary

ACE: a combination chemotherapy regimen containing actinomycin D, cyclophosphamide and etoposide

AFP: α-fetoprotein, a marker for the presence of certain tumours

BEP: a combination chemotherapy regimen containing bleomycin, etoposide and cisplatin

CT: computed tomography

FSH: follicle-stimulating hormone, a gonadotrophic hormone secreted by the pituitary gland

GnRH: gonadotrophin-releasing hormone, a hormone that controls the release of FSH and LH; it is secreted by the hypothalamus

hCG: human chorionic gonadotrophin, a hormone that helps to maintain early pregnancy. It also serves as a tumour marker

ICSI: intracytoplasmic sperm injection, a technique in which a single sperm is injected into a processed egg

LH: luteinizing hormone, a gonadotrophic hormone secreted by the pituitary gland

MESA: microscopic epididymal sperm aspiration

MRI: magnetic resonance imaging

PESA: percutaneous epididymal sperm aspiration

POMB: a combination chemotherapy regimen containing cisplatin, vincristine, methotrexate and bleomycin

RPLND: retroperitoneal lymph node dissection

SHBG: sex hormone-binding globulin

FAST FACTS

the Testis

Timothy J Christmas
Consultant Urological Surgeon,
Charing Cross and Chelsea & Westminster
Hospitals, London, UK

Michael D Dinneen
Consultant Urological Surgeon,
Charing Cross and Chelsea & Westminster
Hospitals, London, UK

Larry Lipshultz
Professor of Urology,
Scott Department of Urology, Baylor College
of Medicine, Houston, Texas, USA

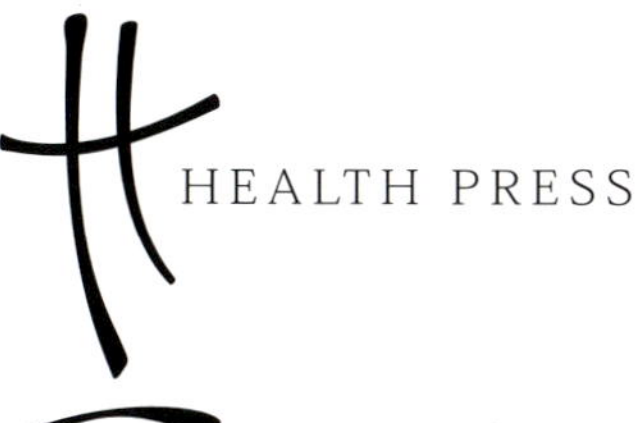

Oxford

Fast Facts – Diseases of the Testis
First published 1999

Elizabeth House, Queen Street, Abingdon, Oxford, OX14 3JR, UK
Tel: +44 (0)1235 523233
Fax: +44 (0)1235 523238

A CIP catalogue record for this title is available from the British Library.

ISBN 1-899541-46-2

Library of Congress
Cataloguing-in-Publication Data

Christmas, TJ (Timothy)
Fast Facts – Diseases of the Testis/
Timothy J Christmas, Michael D Dinneen,
Larry Lipshultz

Illustrated by MeDee Art, London, UK

Printed by Fine Print, Oxford, UK

Introduction

A wide range of disorders can affect the testes, the scrotal skin and other scrotal contents. *Fast Facts – Diseases of the Testis* provides a comprehensive but concise description of congenital conditions, acquired benign disorders, infections of the scrotal contents, malignant diseases and the investigation and treatment of male infertility.

The increasing interest in the field of testicular disease stems from recent reports that the incidences of cryptorchidism and testicular cancer are increasing, and that men's sperm counts are declining. Could this be a congenital or environmental phenomenon? Is environmental radiation or pollution from the oestrogens used in animal feeds leading to a decline in male fertility and an increase in testicular cancer? These questions cannot yet be answered with certainty. However, male infertility is now a discrete sub-specialty and major advances have been made, enabling men with even the lowest level of sperm production to father children.

Cancer of the testis is the most common malignancy in young men. Its treatment is a shining example of successful modern oncological practice, with cure rates for metastatic disease exceeding 90% in major cancer centres.

These topical issues are discussed in *Fast Facts – Diseases of the Testis*. The structured text and tables are complemented by clinical pictures and diagrams. We hope that this short book will be a useful reference work for family physicians, trainee urologists, gynaecologists, genitourinary physicians and nurses.

CHAPTER 1

Anatomy and physiology

The human testis is a paired organ that is normally found in the scrotum. The testis has two main functions:

- spermatogenesis, which occurs in the seminiferous tubules
- secretion of the male hormones (androgens) by the Leydig cells found in the interstitial tissue between the seminiferous tubules.

Anatomy

The scrotum consists of corrugated skin, under which is found the dartos muscle. Contraction of this muscle contributes to testicular temperature regulation. Deep to this muscle are three fascial layers derived from the layers of the abdominal wall – the intracolumnar fascia, the cremasteric fascia and the infundibuliform fascia. The testis is covered anteriorly and laterally by the visceral layer of the tunica vaginalis, which is continuous with its parietal layer, and superficial to this are the fascial layers of scrotal wall (Figure 1.1).

Figure 1.1 Transverse section through the scrotum.

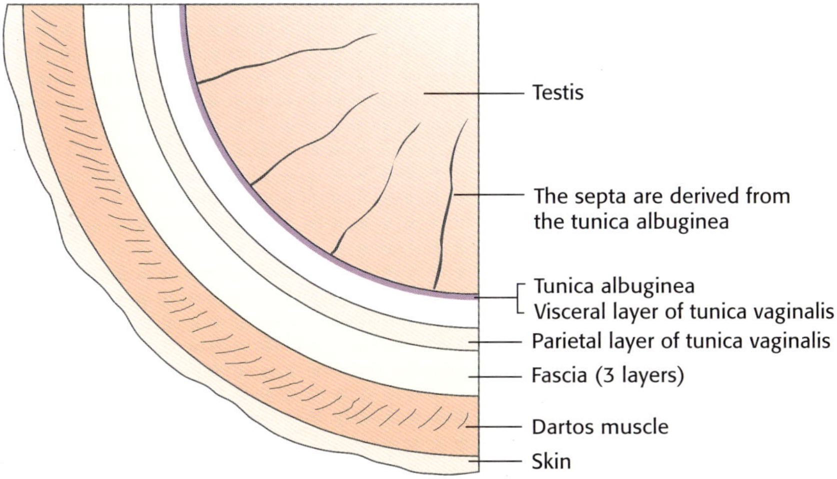

A midline septum of connective tissue divides the scrotum into two sacs, which contain the two testes (Figure 1.2). The average adult testis weighs around 25 g and measures 4 x 5 x 2.5 cm. It is covered by a dense white fascia, the tunica albuginea, which indents the testis posteriorly (rete testis) and sends fibrous septa into the body of the testis to form about 250 lobules. The appendix testis is a small pedunculated or sessile body found at the upper pole of the testis. Posterolateral to the testis is the epididymis, which at its upper pole is attached to the body of the testis by numerous ducts. The epididymis consists of a coiled duct, forming at its lower pole the vas deferens, which lies behind and medial to the testis.

Figure 1.2 The testis.

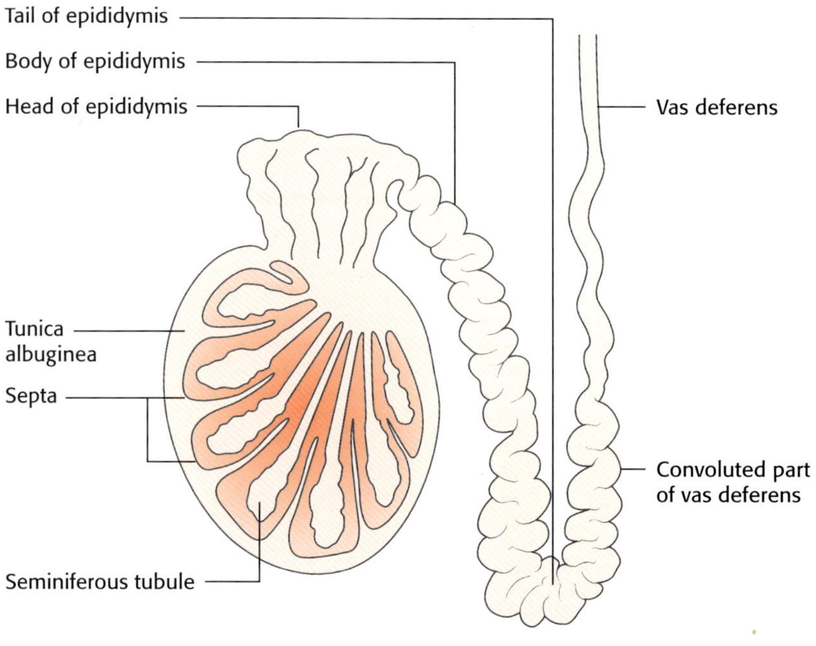

Histology

Each testicular lobule contains between one and four convoluted seminiferous tubules, each of which is about 60 cm in length. The tubules converge at the rete testis, where they coalesce to form the efferent ducts that empty into the epididymis. Each seminiferous tubule is lined by a basement membrane of connective tissue, which supports the two types of seminiferous cells, the supporting or Sertoli cells, and the germ cells at various stages of maturation (Figure 1.3).

The Sertoli cells are non-dividing and help to form the blood–testis barrier. In addition to providing nourishment for the germ cells and removing effete cells by phagocytosis, this barrier maintains an immunologically privileged location around the germ cells.

The germ cells are arranged from the basement membrane to the lumen of the seminiferous tubules in an orderly manner from least to most differentiated. The most primitive or stem cells are called spermatogonia; these divide and differentiate through spermatocytes and spermatids to ultimately become spermatozoa. Sperm are produced in the testis but maturation occurs in the epididymis.

Embryology

Embryos are initially bisexual. Male and female potentials are represented in the sexually undifferentiated gonad – normal sexual differentiation involves gradual predominance of one component. Primitive gonads first appear on the urogenital ridge during the fifth and sixth weeks. During the seventh week, differentiation into testis or ovary begins. Adjacent to the primitive gonad lie the nephric (Wolffian) and Müllerian ducts. The former is

Figure 1.3 Transverse section of the seminiferous tubule (approximately x500).

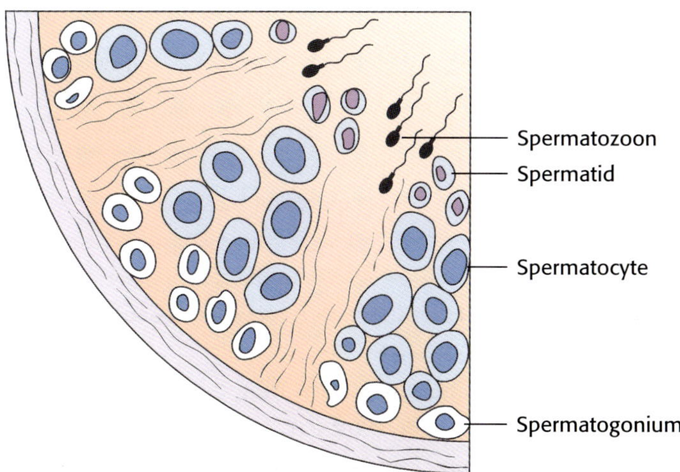

important in the development of the urinary tract and the male genital tract, while the latter is primarily a female genital structure from the start. The Wolffian duct forms the middle and terminal portion of the epididymis, vas deferens, seminal vesicles and ejaculatory ducts. The Müllerian duct regresses in the male, with only its upper and lower portions remaining as the appendix testis and as a portion of the prostatic utricle, respectively. The lumina of the mesonephric tubules at the head end of the Wolffian duct become continuous with those of the rete testis to form the caput epididymis. The adjacent lower part of the Wolffian duct forms the vas deferens.

During the sixth week, the gonad consists of a superficial germinal epithelium and an internal blastema. In the male, the cells of this epithelium grow into the blastema to form cord-like masses; these are radially arranged and converge towards the attachments to the Wolffian duct to form a gonadal mesentery known as the mesorchium. These cords become differentiated into the seminiferous tubules.

During the twelfth week, the testis is located retroperitoneally. A fibromuscular band (gubernaculum testis) extends from the lower pole of the testis through the muscular layers of the anterior abdominal wall to end in the subcutaneous tissues of the developing scrotum. A peritoneal herniation (the processus vaginalis) accompanies the testis to the scrotum. The testis remains close to the internal ring of the inguinal canal until the seventh month, and normally reaches the scrotal sac by the end of the eighth month (Figure 1.4).

Physiology

The anterior pituitary gland controls testicular sperm and hormone production by the testis, through the secretion of the gonadotrophins follicle-stimulating hormone (FSH) and luteinizing hormone (LH), respectively. The release of FSH and LH is controlled by the secretion of gonadotrophin-releasing hormone (GnRH) by the hypothalamus. GnRH secretion, in turn, is controlled by higher centres in the central nervous system and by negative feedback (a closed-loop feedback mechanism) from the testis (Figure 1.5).

Testosterone is secreted intermittently by the Leydig cells under the control of LH, and levels vary throughout the day. Normally only 2% of testosterone is free, 44% is bound by sex hormone-binding globulin

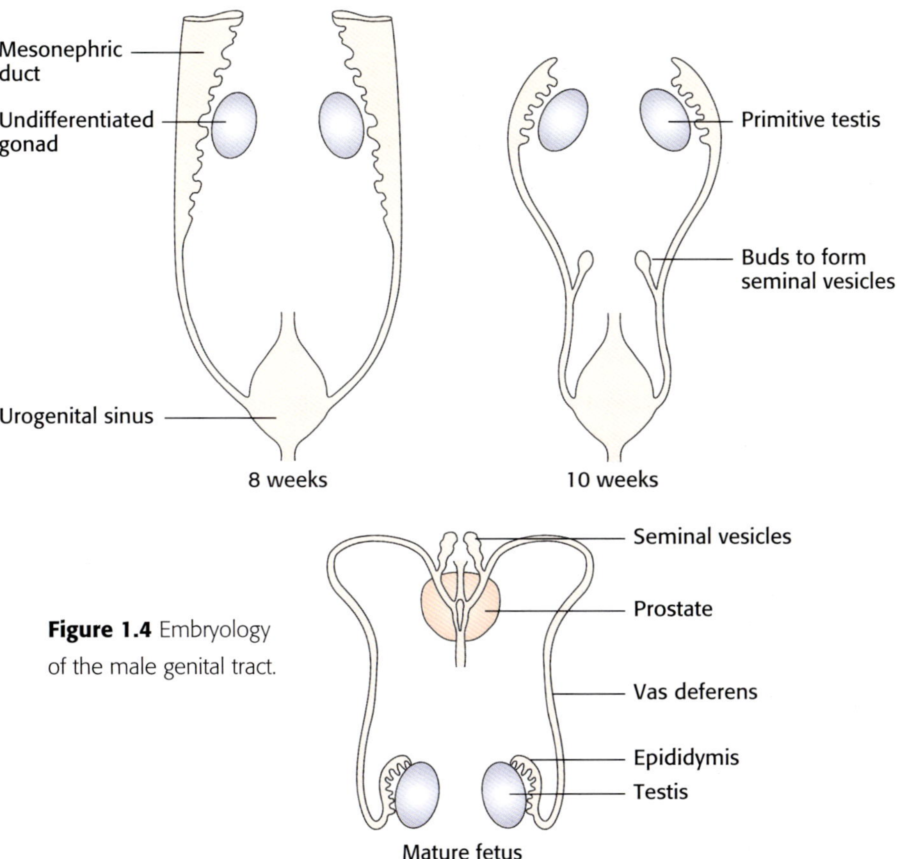

Figure 1.4 Embryology of the male genital tract.

(SHBG), and the remainder is bound to other proteins, including albumin. Many factors can influence the levels of SHBG, and thus also influence the activity of testosterone (Table 1.1). Elevation in SHBG levels reduces the amount of free testosterone available for metabolism, thus the plasma

TABLE 1.1

Factors that affect plasma SHBG levels

Plasma SHBG decreased by:	Plasma SHBG increased by:
• Androgen therapy	• Oestrogen therapy
• Growth hormone therapy	• Thyroxine therapy
• Obesity	• Cirrhosis

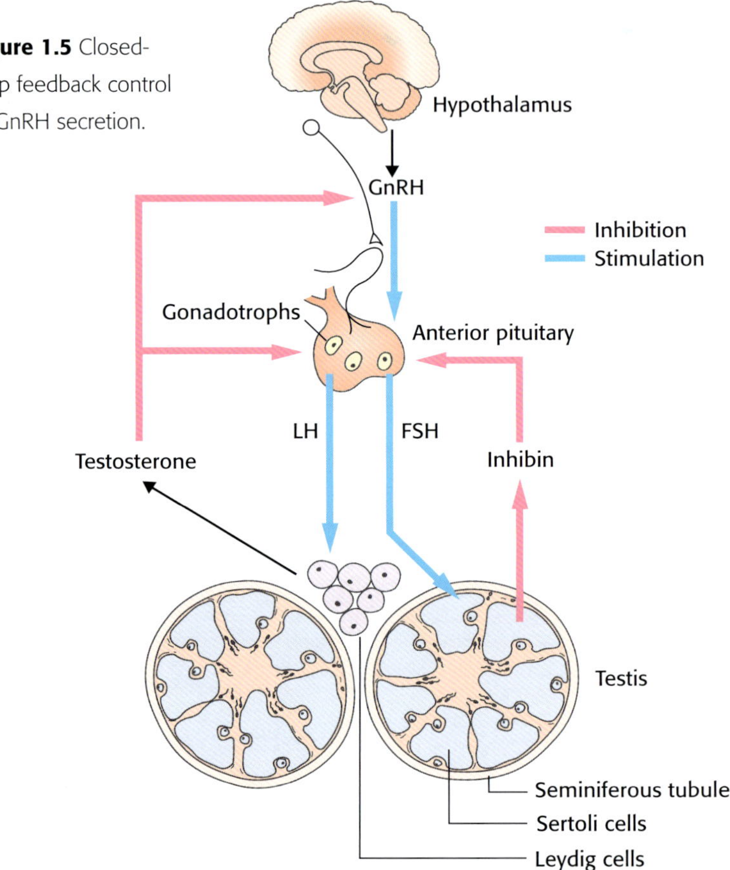

Figure 1.5 Closed-loop feedback control of GnRH secretion.

concentration of SHBG is inversely related to the activity of testosterone. The exact physiological role of SHBG in man is not known. The main functions of testosterone and its breakdown products are listed in Table 1.2.

TABLE 1.2

The main functions of testosterone and its breakdown products

- Initiation of spermatogenesis
- Maintenance of spermatogenesis
- Control of gonadotrophin secretion by the hypothalamic–pituitary axis
- Male differentiation during fetal development
- Sexual maturation at puberty

CHAPTER 2

Congenital anomalies

Anomalies of number

True absence of one or both testes is extremely rare. A careful search must be conducted for an impalpable testis. All the modern imaging techniques may be of use, and in particular:

- selective gonadal venography
- ultrasonography
- computed tomographic (CT) scanning
- laparoscopy
- magnetic resonance imaging (MRI).

Similarly, the presence of more than two testes is very rare, and the differential diagnosis includes:

- hydrocele of the cord
- spermatocele
- epididymal cysts.

Hypogonadism

This section is confined to the discussion of phenotypic (46, XY) males presenting with a delay in the onset of puberty. The clinical features are listed in Table 2.1 and possible causes of delayed puberty in Table 2.2.

TABLE 2.1

A number of clinical features should lead the family physician to suspect the presence of hypogonadism

- Lack of erections, nocturnal emissions and decreased libido
- Absence of pubic, axillary and facial hair
- Juvenile voice persisting
- Sitting to standing height ratio < 1:2
- Small penis and scrotum
- Small or absent testes

TABLE 2.2

Delayed puberty may have no obvious cause or be the result of either hypergonadotrophic hypogonadism or hypogonadotrophic hypogonadism, for each of which there are several possible causes

Idiopathic	
Hypergonadotrophic hypogonadism	• Congenital anorchia • Acquired anorchia • Klinefelter's syndrome
Hypogonadotrophic hypogonadism	• Pituitary tumours • Cerebral irradiation • Meningitis • Trauma • Rare syndromes, e.g. Kallmann's or Prader-Willi syndrome

- Idiopathic or constitutional delay is the most common cause for the late onset of secondary sexual characteristics, and there is often a family history. The diagnosis is largely clinical, and the treatment is based on counselling and support.
- In hypergonadotrophic hypogonadism, basal levels of both FSH and LH are raised, and there is an exaggerated response to GnRH.
- In hypogonadotrophic hypogonadism, FSH and LH levels are low, but the response to GnRH depends on whether the defect lies in the pituitary gland or the hypothalamus.

Specific treatment of hypogonadism depends on the cause, but is largely based on the administration of exogenous testosterone. Four different methods are currently in use:

- tablets
- patches
- intramuscular injections
- subcutaneous implants.

Although oral testosterone is easy to take, its clinical efficacy is, at best, variable. Testosterone patches are reported to provide physiological levels, but local skin reactions may occur. Intramuscular injections are uncomfortable and the treatment regimen requires regular visits to the clinic (3–4-weekly). Implants are usually effective for 6 months and have few side-effects.

Ectopy and cryptorchidism

Epidemiology and pathophysiology. Cryptorchidism is the most common malformation of an endocrine gland in the male population. The prevalence of cryptorchidism in term infants is 3–4%, whereas the prevalence at 1 year of age is 0.8%. Spontaneous descent of a truly cryptorchid testis seldom occurs after the first year of life. Normal testicular descent appears to be due to a combination of mechanical and hormonal factors, which are poorly understood in the human. Beginning at the end of the first year of life, the undescended testis undergoes progressive histological deterioration compared with a normal testis. The more severe the malposition of the undescended testis, the greater the degree of histological damage.

A cryptorchid testis may also descend to an ectopic site (i.e. one other than the scrotal sac). Possible ectopic sites are listed in Table 2.3.

Cryptorchid testes have a 40-times greater risk of developing a germ cell tumour than a scrotal testis, have lower sperm densities, and have a greater risk of undergoing testicular torsion. In addition, 95% are associated with a patent processus vaginalis (25% are associated with a detectable inguinal hernia).

TABLE 2.3

Ectopic sites

Ectopic site	Frequency
Superficial inguinal	Most common
Perineal	Rare
Femoral	Rare
Penile	Rare
Paradoxical (both testes in same inguinal canal)	Rare
Pelvic	Rare

Diagnosis. Cryptorchidism is characterized by the absence of the testis from the scrotum. The older patient may complain of pain from a testis in an abnormal position. Occasionally a patient with bilateral undescended testes may present with infertility. On examination the ipsilateral hemiscrotum may be underdeveloped and an indirect inguinal hernia may be present. If both testes are absent, a human chorionic gonadotrophin (hCG) test may establish the presence of testosterone-producing tissue. Ultrasonographic examination may help to locate a testis in the groin, but is less useful with intra-abdominal testes. CT scanning, MRI and selective gonadal venography may all be of benefit. Laparoscopy will ultimately identify an intra-abdominal testis or confirm the absence or presence of gonadal vessels entering the internal inguinal ring.

A retractile testis is one that is pulled out of the scrotum by an overactive cremaster muscle. There may be a history of the testis having been descended at the time of a previous examination and the experienced examiner can usually manipulate such a testis into the scrotum.

Management. Controversy exists about hormonal therapy for undescended testes. Treatment with hCG or GnRH has been shown to be successful within about 1 month in 10–20% of cases, with more success in bilateral cryptorchidism than in unilateral cryptorchidism.

The gold standard for treatment remains surgical orchidopexy (Figure 2.1). The basic principles are:

- identification and mobilization of the testis and spermatic cord to allow placement of the testis in the dependent part of the ipsilateral hemiscrotum without tension
- repair of any associated hernia.

Complications of this procedure are unusual, but include damage to the vas deferens, damage to the ilioinguinal nerve, retraction of the testis due to inadequate dissection of the cord and testicular atrophy due to vascular damage.

Techniques for placing high or intra-abdominal testes in the scrotum include:

- the single-stage or two-stage Fowler-Stephen's technique
- staged orchidopexy
- microvascular autotransplantation.

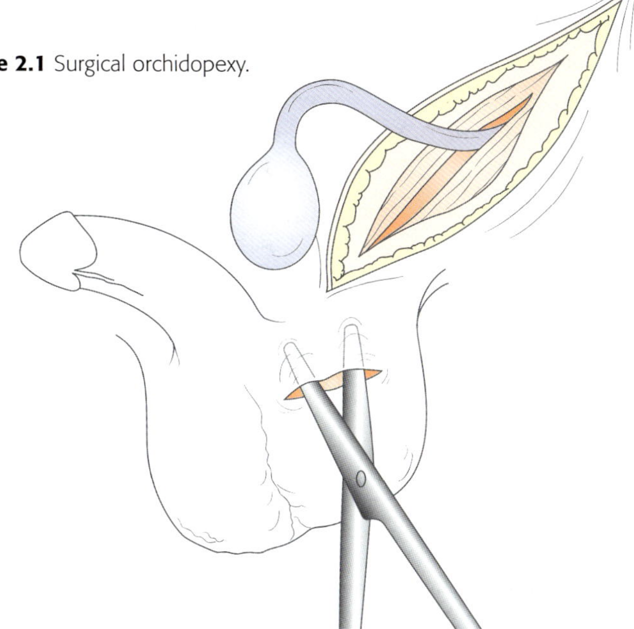

Figure 2.1 Surgical orchidopexy.

Intersex

The chromosomal make-up of an individual (i.e. the genotype, XX or XY) determines which gonad (either testis or ovary) is formed. This in turn controls the development of the respective male or female genital tracts (i.e. the phenotype), and the ability to reproduce. Any disturbance in this process may lead to abnormalities in sexual differentiation, the so-called 'intersex' group of disorders.

Full discussion of intersex is beyond the scope of this text, but they can be broadly grouped into four simplified categories.

Female pseudohermaphroditism (XX). Ovaries, uterus and Fallopian tubes are normal, but external genitalia are male. The most common causes are congenital adrenal hyperplasia and maternal virilizing syndromes. It is, therefore, a phenotypic disorder.

Male pseudohermaphroditism (XY). Virilization of the male embryo is defective, mostly due to defects in androgen synthesis or action. This is also a phenotypic disorder – patients with mild hypospadias or a single undescended testis fall at the least affected end of the spectrum.

True hermaphroditism (XX, XY or mosaic). In this rare condition, both ovaries and testes are present. This disorder occurs at the chromosomal level.

Gonadal dysgenesis (Turner's syndrome). This condition is characterized by female phenotype but primary amenorrhoea, infertility and streak gonads. It is a chromosomal disorder, with the most common abnormality being a single X chromosome.

Diagnosis. This depends on a full family history and careful physical examination, followed by the establishment of the chromosomal sex. In some cases, biochemical, endoscopic and radiological evaluation may be required. Rarely, exploratory laparotomy may also be needed. The presence of a hypospadiac meatus in association with either unilateral or bilateral cryptorchidism should alert the examiner to a possible intersex state. If the external genitalia are ambiguous and cryptorchidism and hypospadias are present, the incidence of intersex is approximately 50%. If the external genitalia are normal in the presence of the other abnormalities, the risk of intersex falls to 25%.

Management. In all patients with ambiguous genitalia, the main goal must be to establish a diagnosis and to assign a sex for rearing that is compatible with a well-adjusted life and sexual adequacy. Often the major factor in recommending male sex assignment is an adequate size and a potential for development of the penis.

Once the sex for rearing has been decided, it is important that the gender role is reinforced by surgical means and, most importantly, by hormonal measures.

CHAPTER 3

Infective conditions of the testicle

Inflammation can occur anywhere in the male genitourinary tract – this chapter focuses particularly on epididymitis and orchitis. Severe epididymitis may develop into epididymo-orchitis. Isolated orchitis is much less common.

Epididymitis

Epididymitis, the most common intrascrotal inflammatory condition, may be acute or chronic. Epididymitis may develop following instrumentation of the urinary tract, urinary tract infection, prostatitis, or may arise *de novo*.

Acute epididymitis may be divided into three types:

- non-specific bacterial
- sexually transmitted
- uncommon causes.

Pathophysiology. Non-specific bacterial epididymitis is common in older men, and is usually caused by Gram-negative aerobic rods. It is often associated with underlying urological pathology. The usual route of infection is retrograde ascent from the urethra and prostate via the ejaculatory ducts and vasa deferentia. High intravesical pressures have also been implicated. Haematogenous and lymphatic spread may be important in some cases.

Some common organisms causing sexually transmitted epididymitis are *Chlamydia trachomatis* and *Neisseria gonorrhoeae*, commonly occurring together. There is often an associated urethritis, and this condition is much more common in younger men. Uncommon causes of epididymitis include vasectomy, trauma and tuberculosis.

In most cases of epididymitis, the inflammation spreads from the lower pole of the epididymis to the upper pole, there is often an associated hydrocele, and the testis may become involved (Figure 3.1). The inflammation may resolve without scarring, but fibrosis may develop and obstruct the testicular ducts or epididymis. Acute epididymitis can give rise to a number of complications, which are shown in Table 3.1.

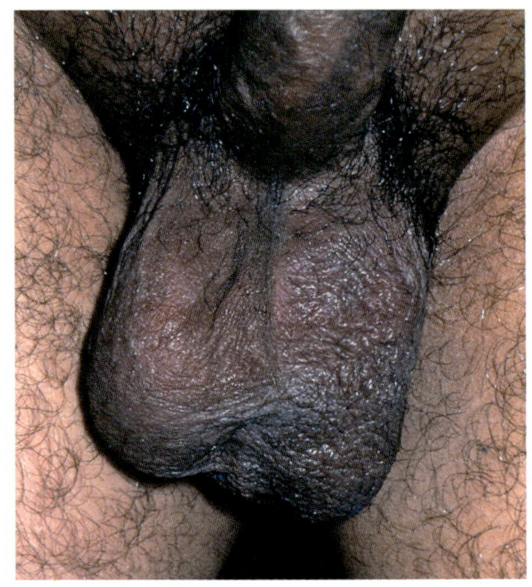

Figure 3.1 Clinical features of epididymitis.

Diagnosis. The epididymis is usually quite tender, and a urethral discharge may be noted. The overlying scrotal skin is reddened, and although early in the illness the epididymis and the testis may be distinguishable, they quickly become one mass. The prostate may also be tender. The investigations that should be undertaken for acute epididymitis are shown in Table 3.2.

If an organism is isolated in the urine, a presumptive diagnosis of epididymitis due to that organism may be made. Care must be taken to exclude other possible diagnoses (Table 3.3), particularly as the presenting symptoms are very similar to those of testicular torsion.

Treatment. General supportive measures, such as bed rest and analgesia, are usually required. More specifically, a scrotal support and ice packs may be of benefit.

The recommended antibacterial treatment is detailed in Table 3.4. In general practice, the recommended treatment for acute epididymitis is a 2–4-week course (depending on the source of the infection) of an oral quinolone, such as ciprofloxacin, which is active against both Gram-positive and Gram-negative organisms in addition to *Chlamydia*. Other

TABLE 3.1

Complications of acute epididymitis

- Testicular infarction
- Scrotal abscess
- Chronic discharging sinus
- Chronic epididymitis
- Infertility

TABLE 3.2

Investigations for acute epididymitis aim to distinguish infective from non-infective causes

- Urethral smear for Gram staining and culture of *Chlamydia* and *Neisseria gonorrhoeae*
- Urinalysis
- Mid-stream urine specimen
- Cultures for sexually transmitted pathogens
- Scrotal colour Doppler ultrasound

antibacterials in this group include norfloxacin, enoxacin and ofloxacin. In addition to its broad spectrum of activity, ciprofloxacin penetrates well into the prostate, testis and epididymis, and reaches higher levels in these tissues than many other antibiotics. Doxycycline may also be used as a standard treatment. With prompt diagnosis and treatment, resolution and recovery are usually complete but may take 4–6 weeks.

In order to reduce the risk of epididymitis developing, it is essential to identify and treat underlying urinary tract infections in patients undergoing any urological procedures.

Chronic epididymitis. This is the irreversible end stage of recurrent acute epididymitis, in which there is induration of the organ due to fibrosis and scarring with tubular occlusion. Lymphocytes and plasma cells are in evidence. The condition causes varying degrees of pain and the epididymis may or may not be tender. An associated pyuria is not uncommon. If chronic

TABLE 3.3

Differential diagnosis of acute epididymitis

- Testicular torsion (see page 25)
- Tumours, painless (see page 31)
- Tuberculous epididymitis – rare, painless
- Torsion of the appendages of the testis (see page 27)
- Trauma

TABLE 3.4

Antimicrobial treatment of acute epididymitis

Sexually transmitted acute epididymitis
• Single intramuscular dose of second- or third-generation cephalosporin plus a 2-week course of an oral tetracycline, OR • A 2–3-week course of an oral quinolone
Non-sexually transmitted acute epididymitis
• Prompt treatment with an appropriate antimicrobial based on culture and sensitivity, OR • A 2–4-week course of an oral quinolone

tuberculous epididymitis is suspected (sterile pyuria, tubercle bacilli in urine, or beading of the vas deferens), intravenous urography is indicated to exclude disease elsewhere in the urinary tract. Treatment is antibiotic based, but extensive scarring may prevent therapeutic levels being reached. Very occasionally, excision of the entire epididymis is required.

Orchitis

Isolated orchitis is much less common than either epididymitis or urethritis. Unlike other genital tract infections, the route of spread of the organism is haematogenous and viruses are important in the aetiology of many cases (Table 3.5).

Differential diagnosis. This is similar to that for acute epididymitis (see Table 3.3). Some urologists recommend surgical exploration for every young man presenting with acute unilateral scrotal pathology to avoid missing a case of testicular torsion. Patients with acute epididymitis, orchitis and epididymo-orchitis must be followed up once the cardinal signs of inflammation have subsided to identify a possible testicular tumour masquerading as an inflammatory condition. Scrotal ultrasound is indicated where there is suspicion of testicular tumour.

Mumps orchitis is the most common of the viral orchitides. It seldom occurs in prepubertal boys, but develops in 20–30% of those who contract the

TABLE 3.5

Classification of orchitis

Viral

- Mumps
- Coxsackie B
- Varicella

Pyogenic (usually associated with epididymitis)

- Gram-negative aerobic rods
- Diphtheria
- Schistosomiasis
- Filariasis
- Amoebiasis

Granulomatous

- Syphilis
- Tuberculosis
- Actinomycosis
- Fungal disease

infection after puberty. Testicular pain and swelling classically occur 4 days following the onset of parotitis, but very occasionally may occur in isolation. The scrotal skin is usually erythematous and oedematous, and urinary symptoms are very occasionally a feature. An acute hydrocele may develop and a high fever may be found.

Treatment is supportive – bed rest, analgesia and scrotal support. Specific measures including steroid therapy have been recommended, but their benefit remains unproven. More recently, the use of immunotherapeutic agents, such as interferon, for the protection of the testes has been reported. About 50% of testes that become clinically involved by mumps after puberty develop some degree of atrophy, which is usually apparent within 2 months. Sterility may result in bilateral cases but is relatively uncommon.

Acute pyogenic orchitis in isolation (without associated epididymitis) is very rare. The clinical course and complications of orchitis are similar to those of epididymitis: the patient is often unwell with a high fever, severe pain, nausea and vomiting. Urine and blood cultures may help to direct specific therapy. Surgical treatment and debridement, including orchidectomy, may be required. Any patient presenting with isolated orchitis should be evaluated for underlying testicular tumour or missed testicular torsion.

Granulomatous orchitis is now rare, but both congenital and acquired syphilis are still seen. Isolated tuberculous orchitis is also rare.

CHAPTER 4

Acquired benign diseases

A variety of benign, non-infective disorders can affect the contents of the scrotum and these are described below. Table 4.1 summarizes the key clinical findings in the differential diagnosis of all swellings within the scrotum.

TABLE 4.1

Differential diagnosis of swellings of the scrotum

	Hydrocele	Epididymal cyst	Inguino-scrotal hernia	Varicocele
Pain	–	–	+ or –	– or minor
Testis separate from mass	–	+	+	+
Hard	–	–	–	–
Reducible	–	–	+ or –	–
Larger when standing	–	–	+	+
Trans-illuminable	+	+	–	–
Testis high in scrotum	–	–	–	–

	Epididymo-orchitis	Testicular cancer	Torsion of the testis
Pain	++	– or minor	+++
Testis separate from mass	–	–	–
Hard	+	++	+
Reducible	–	–	–
Larger when standing	–	–	–
Trans-illuminable	–	–	–
Testis high in scrotum	–	–	+

Torsion of the testis

Epidemiology and pathophysiology. Torsion of the testis most commonly occurs in young males between the ages of 12 and 18 years. Individuals with a narrow testicular mesenteric attachment or a horizontal 'bell-clapper' testis are more likely to develop torsion. Torsion initially leads to swelling of the testis due to venous congestion, which rapidly causes reduction in flow and then complete cessation of arterial input to the affected testis. Torsion should be the initial diagnosis for any patient presenting with acute testicular pain.

Diagnosis. The presenting symptom is pain of acute origin in the affected testis, which becomes enlarged. On examination the entire testis, rather than just the epididymis, is tender and swollen and this factor alone can be used to distinguish torsion from epididymitis. Often the torted testis lies high within the scrotum and there may be a palpable twist in the distal cord (Figure 4.1). Clinical diagnosis is generally all that is required before planning treatment. If there is doubt over the diagnosis, however, either colour Doppler ultrasonography or radioimmunoscintigraphy can be used to show a reduced blood supply to the testis caused by twisting of the cord.

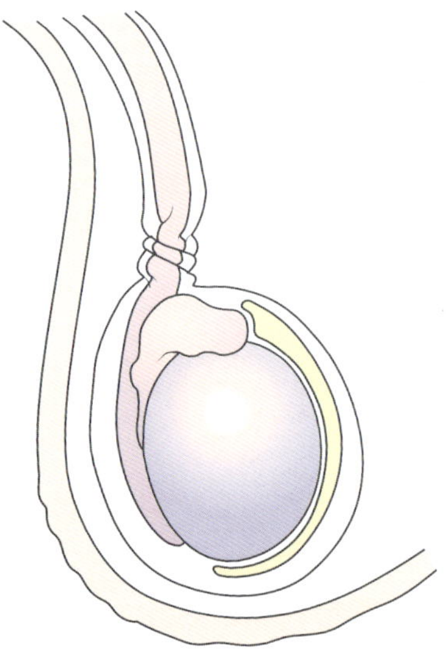

Figure 4.1 Torsion of the testis. The twist in the torted testis may be palpable.

Management. Early surgical intervention is mandatory. The affected testis is explored through a midline scrotal incision and is usually found to be dusky blue in colour. Initially the testis is untwisted and examined after a few minutes to determine whether recovery is feasible. If the testis remains dusky in colour and is clearly non-viable, orchidectomy should be performed. If viable, the testis should be fixed to the dartos muscle of the scrotal wall. As the contralateral testis is at increased risk of later torsion, it should also be fixed at the same time. If orchidectomy is necessary, a testicular prosthesis can be inserted at the same time or later (these are not currently available in the USA).

Torsion of the appendix of the testis

The appendix of the testis may undergo torsion and present with acute pain within the scrotum in adolescent boys. Examination reveals a small tender swelling at the upper pole of the testis (Figure 4.2). The presence of the 'blue dot' on trans-illumination is typical. Although conservative management is sometimes successful, surgical excision of the appendix testis may become necessary if pain persists.

Inguino-scrotal hernia

Pathophysiology. These hernias may extend into the scrotum (Figure 4.3) and are most commonly found in young boys and older men. In the former, the hernia may result from a congenital persistence of the processus vaginalis communicating with the peritoneal cavity. In the older age group, there may be an indirect inguinal hernia; a sliding hernia, where the sac lies alongside a segment of bowel, is also a common finding.

The hernial sac may be empty but sometimes contains small intestine, sigmoid colon on the left, or caecum and appendix on the right. Part of the bladder is contained in inguino-scrotal hernias in up to 10% of cases. Very occasionally the distal ureter may also be contained within the hernia. There is a definite risk of strangulation with these hernias, and this is most likely to occur when there is a small hernial opening.

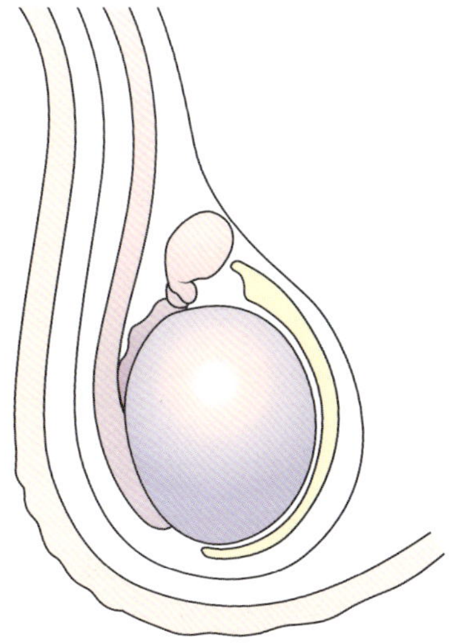

Figure 4.2 Torsion of the appendix of the testis. A small swelling at the upper pole of the testis is usually palpable.

Diagnosis. Inguino-scrotal hernias are painless except when strangulated. Examination reveals a soft mass separate from the testis, which is not trans-illuminable. In most cases the mass can be reduced back into the peritoneal cavity. The hernia may be more prominent when the patient stands up, and in those with larger hernias peristaltic waves emanating from the intestine within the hernia may be visible. Clinical examination is all that is required to establish the diagnosis.

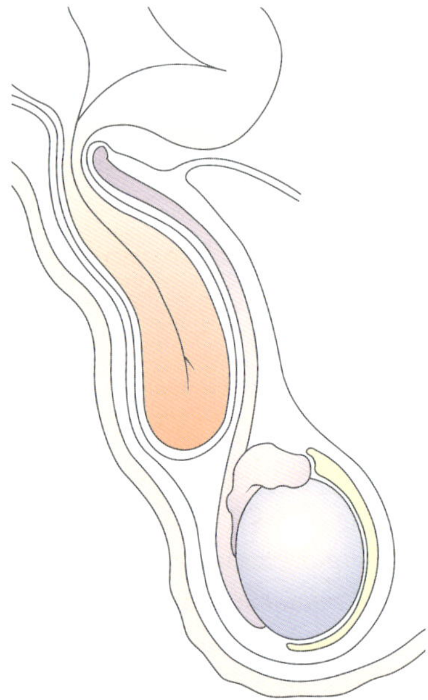

Figure 4.3 An inguino-scrotal hernia extends into the scrotum, and examination reveals a soft mass separate from the testis.

Management. Strangulation may cause intestinal obstruction, which may be accompanied by ischaemia of segments within the sac. This is a life-threatening condition, particularly in elderly men. These potential complications, as well as the symptoms caused by these hernias, have led to the recommendation that, in most circumstances, surgical repair is indicated. Under local or general anaesthesia, a groin incision is made and the hernial contents reduced into the peritoneal cavity. This is more technically demanding with sliding hernias. The hernia defect is repaired: the current vogue is for the Lichtenstein repair, which uses non-absorbable mesh to close the posterior wall of the inguinal canal without tension. In most cases this procedure can be performed as a day case.

Epididymal cyst or spermatocele

Cysts of the epididymis (Figure 4.4) are very common and almost without exception are benign. They may be detected in over 50% of all men on ultrasonography of the scrotum. The cysts are almost always painless and are often multiple. Most are palpable within the epididymis separate from the testis and can be trans-illuminated. Scrotal ultrasonography will confirm the diagnosis.

Management. As most of these cysts are asymptomatic, treatment is usually not necessary. Needle aspiration may be painful and lead to infection, and almost invariably the cyst fluid re-accumulates within 2–3 months.

Injection of sclerosing agents is also painful, and the cyst may recur. In cases in which the cyst causes discomfort or increases to a large size, surgical excision may be indicated. Under local or general anaesthesia, an incision is made directly over the cyst, which is carefully excised. Injudicious dissection of the epididymis may be complicated by damage to tubules with consequent obstruction to the flow of sperm.

Varicocele

Pathophysiology. Dilatation and varicosity of the testicular veins can lead to swelling within the scrotum, referred to as a varicocele (Figure 4.5). This tortuous collection of veins is found on the left side of the scrotum in 90% of cases, and may be bilateral in 30–50%. The aetiology is thought to be a defect in the anti-reflux valves within testicular veins, analogous to varicose veins in the leg, and the increased incidence of left-sided varicoceles relates to the anatomy of the venous system. On the left, the testicular venous drainage is into the left renal vein, while on the right the vein is shorter and there is direct drainage into the inferior vena cava. Varicoceles may lead to a reduction in the sperm count and motility as a result of the rise in scrotal temperature caused by increased blood flow in the veins.

Figure 4.4 Epididymal cysts are usually palpable within the epididymis separate from the testis.

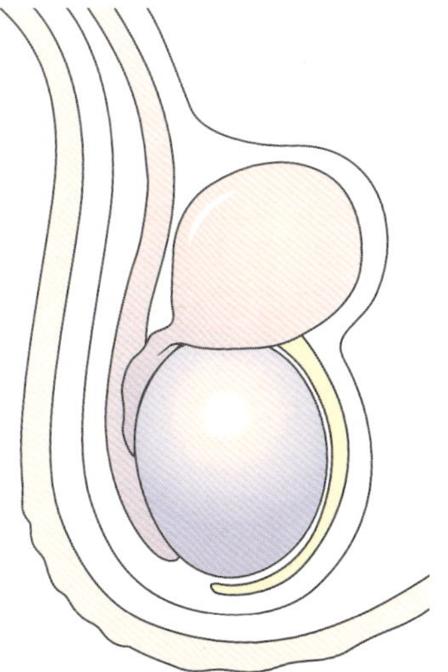

Diagnosis. Fifteen per cent of the normal population have a varicocele. Although many varicoceles are asymptomatic, they may cause discomfort, particularly after prolonged periods of standing, and significant swelling. Varicoceles may be detected during investigation of infertility, and up to 40% of infertile males have a varicocele. They are usually palpable within the scrotum separate from the testis, feel like a ‘bag of worms’, and are more prominent when the patient stands up. Palpation of the testicular (spermatic) cord while the patient performs the Valsalva manoeuvre will reveal an increase in the thickness of the cord or the presence of a discrete pulse due to venous reflux. The diagnosis can be confirmed by scrotal Doppler ultrasound. Thermography of the scrotum will show a rise in scrotal temperature in many cases.

The onset of an isolated varicocele in older men should alert the clinician to the possibility of renal tumour with tumour thrombosis within the renal vein. Ultrasonography of the kidney should detect a renal tumour in such cases. Bulky retroperitoneal tumours or lymph nodes may also cause a varicocele. Detection may require a CT scan.

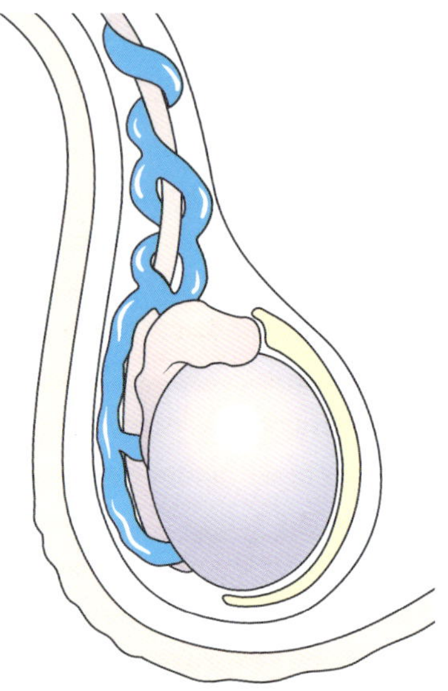

Figure 4.5 Varicoceles are usually palpable within the scrotum separate from the testis, and feel like a 'bag of worms'.

Management. Not all varicoceles need to be treated, but those that should include large varicoceles, those causing significant pain, and those in men with associated suboptimal sperm analysis. The choice of treatment lies between embolization under local anaesthesia by a radiologist, or surgical ligation of the testicular veins. The more minimally invasive radiological technique is successful in many patients, but in the authors' experience incomplete embolization is quite common, as is loin pain after this treatment. In our hands, testicular vein ligation through a retroperitoneal Palomo incision under general anaesthesia has proved to be a successful treatment with a low recurrence rate. Others have described microsurgical inguinal vein ligation with improved presentation of the testicular artery and lymphatic system.

Many studies have shown improvement in semen parameters following varicocele ligation, with some also showing associated increased pregnancy rates.

CHAPTER 5

Tumours of the testis

The peak incidence of cancer of the testis is between the ages of 20 and 40 years, and it is the most common malignant tumour in men within this age group. Over the last 20 years, there has been a steady increase in the incidence of testicular tumours. Established aetiological factors for cancer of the testis include cryptorchidism, atrophy and a history of inguinal hernia repair.

Pathology

The pathological definition of testicular tumours is complex and controversial. Several different classifications have been proposed, but for the sake of uniformity it is best to use the current WHO system as shown in Table 5.1.

It is important to recognize that tumours may be mixed: up to 15% of testicular tumours contain elements of both teratoma and seminoma. Teratomas display embryonic-like characteristics with a variety of tissue elements, which are often inhomogeneous. Seminomas retain the morphology of spermatogonial germ cells and are usually homogeneous. The most common tumour is the testicular teratoma, closely followed by seminoma. A number of rare testicular tumours are not included in Table 5.1, including:

- Leydig cell tumours
- Sertoli cell tumours
- carcinoid tumours
- lymphomas.

Lymphomas are found more often in older patients than in younger ones.

Presentation

The majority of male germ cell tumours arise from the testis. In a small number of cases, germ cell tumours arise from:

- the retroperitoneum
- the anterior mediastinum
- the presacral region
- an area adjacent to the hypothalamus.

Primary testicular tumours most commonly present as a firm, painless enlarging mass within the testis. Unfortunately, the diagnosis is often delayed due to a number of factors, including:

- patient delaying presentation
- misdiagnosis due to pain within the testis, suggesting a possible infective or traumatic aetiology, or even torsion of the testis.

Testicular tumours may occasionally present initially with manifestations distant from the testis. Secretion of hCG by testicular teratomas can lead to gynaecomastia, and it is most important to examine carefully the testes of all men presenting with this condition. Testicular cancer may present with metastatic disease leading to an abdominal mass, enlarged lymph nodes in the neck, pulmonary symptoms, or even neurological symptoms secondary to brain metastases.

TABLE 5.1

WHO pathological classification of testicular tumours

Precursor lesions

- Carcinoma *in situ*

Tumours of one histological type

- Seminoma
- Spermatocytic seminoma
- Embryonal carcinoma
- Yolk sac tumour
- Polyembryoma
- Trophoblastic tumours
  - choriocarcinoma
  - pure
  - mixed
  - placental site implantation tumour

Teratoma

- Mature teratoma
- Immature teratoma
- Teratoma with malignant areas

Mixed tumours of more than one histological type

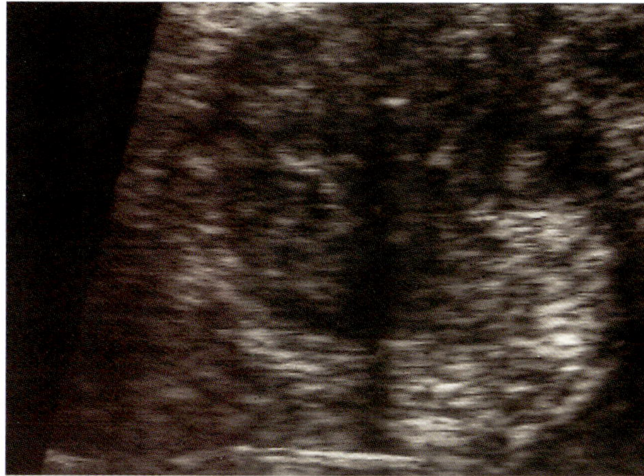

Figure 5.1 Ultrasound scan of the testis showing a cystic teratoma.

Diagnosis

Examination reveals a firm mass within the testis, which is sometimes tender. Ultrasonography of the testis (Figure 5.1) will help to confirm the diagnosis, especially in the presence of a hydrocele. Elevation of the serum testicular tumour markers hCG and α-fetoprotein (AFP) is highly suggestive of the diagnosis of testicular cancer, particularly teratoma. Human chorionic gonadotrophin is produced by syncytiotrophoblasts within teratomas or pure choriocarcinomas, while AFP elevation suggests the presence of yolk sac elements within the tumour. It is important in all but the most extreme cases of high-volume metastatic disease to confirm the diagnosis by inguinal radical orchidectomy initially (Figures 5.2 and 5.3).

Radical orchidectomy should be performed through an inguinal incision. At first, the internal inguinal ring is exposed and the spermatic cord is initially controlled with a soft clamp to prevent dissemination of tumour during mobilization of the testis. The testis is lifted out of the scrotum and dissected free from the scrotal skin by division of the gubernaculum. In most cases, the clinical diagnosis will be sufficiently certain to proceed with radical orchidectomy. If there is any doubt, however, a biopsy should be taken and subjected to immediate frozen section examination. The spermatic cord is ligated and the testis removed. Some patients may request insertion of a testicular prosthesis, and this can be placed within the scrotum via the inguinal incision after orchidectomy (Figure 5.4). The inguinal wound is closed with absorbable sutures.

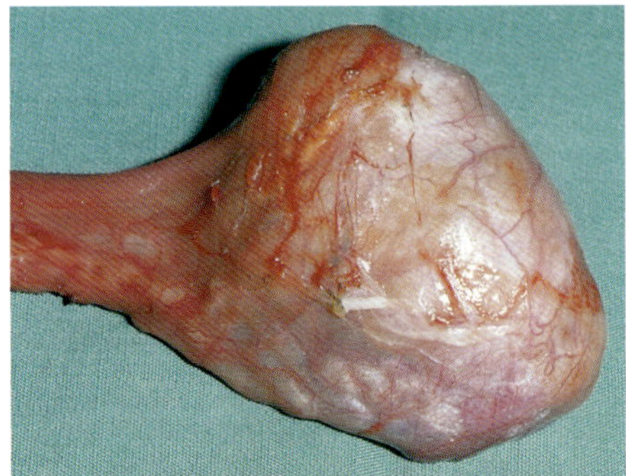

Figure 5.2 Orchidectomy specimen showing irregularity of the tunica albuginea due to a teratoma within the testis.

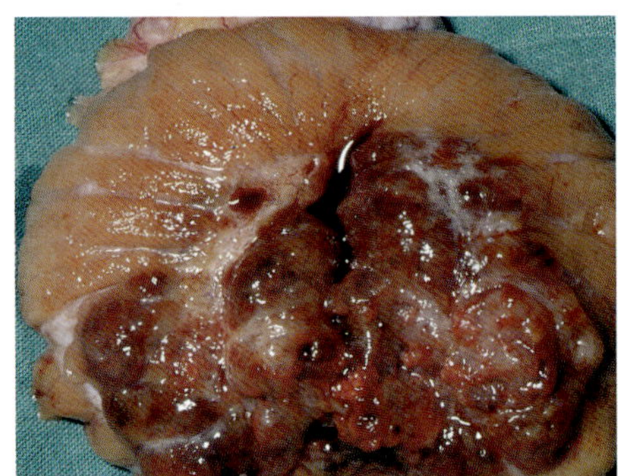

Figure 5.3 The testis has been bivalved to show an inhomogeneous testicular teratoma – the red areas contain choriocarcinomatous elements.

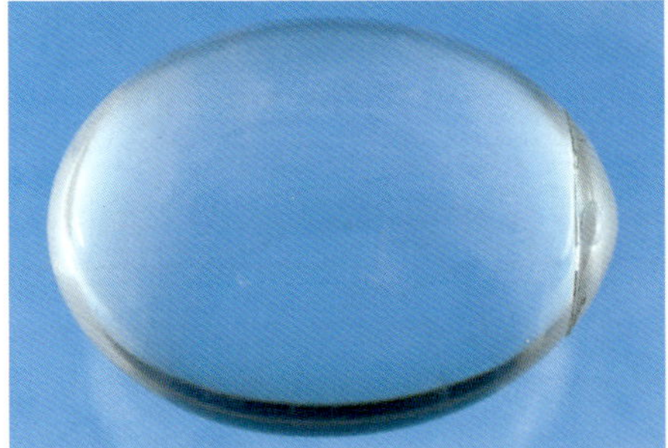

Figure 5.4 Testicular prosthesis – this should be placed into the scrotum through an inguinal incision.

Staging

While the patient is under general anaesthesia for his orchidectomy, deep palpation of the abdomen may reveal nodal metastases within the para-aortic lymph nodes. After orchidectomy, an abdominal CT or MRI scan is essential to stage the disease before planning further treatment. The most common site for metastatic disease is the para-aortic lymph nodes ipsilateral to the primary tumour. In more advanced stages, however, it is not uncommon for lung metastases to be evident. One of several staging systems is shown in Table 5.2.

TABLE 5.2

Royal Marsden Hospital staging for testicular cancer

Stage		Definition
I		No evidence of metastases
	M	Rising markers without other evidence of metastases
II		Abdominal nodal metastases
	A	< 2 cm in diameter
	B	2–5 cm in diameter
	C	> 5 cm in diameter
III		Supra-diaphragmatic nodal metastases
	M	Mediastinal
	N	Supra-clavicular, cervical or axillary
	O	No abdominal disease
IV		Extra-lymphatic metastases
	L1	< 3 lung metastases
	L2	> 3 lung metastases, all < 2 cm in diameter
	L3	> 3 lung metastases, one or more > 2 cm in diameter
	H+	Liver metastases
	Br+	Brain metastases
	Bo+	Bone metastases

Management

In stage I disease radical orchidectomy alone may be sufficient to cure the disease, but long-term follow-up by clinical examination, scanning and tumour marker assay is essential for all patients. In some centres, seminomas are treated with a post-orchidectomy course of radiation to the retroperitoneum, although this is becoming less popular due to potential late side-effects. In the USA and some European countries, it is common practice to perform retroperitoneal lymph node dissection (RPLND) in patients with clinical stage I testicular teratoma, even though metastases are seldom found within the excised lymph nodes.

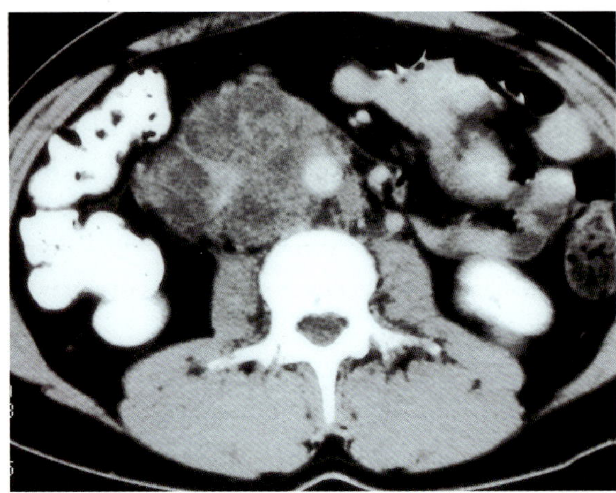

Figure 5.5 Abdominal CT scan showing a mass of lymph nodes containing metastatic disease arising from a right-sided testicular teratoma. The nodes are encasing the inferior vena cava and part of the abdominal aorta.

When there is evidence of metastatic disease on CT scanning (Figure 5.5), with or without elevation of tumour markers after orchidectomy, the initial treatment of choice is usually chemotherapy. Metastatic testicular teratoma is highly sensitive to platinum-based chemotherapy regimens (Figure 5.6), which are the initial treatments of choice for stage II–IV disease. At Charing Cross Hospital, we favour an intensive course of alternating cisplatin, vincristine, methotrexate, bleomycin (POMB) and actinomycin D, cyclophosphamide, etoposide (ACE). For small-volume disease, an intensive regimen of bleomycin, etoposide and cisplatin (BEP) is another therapeutic option.

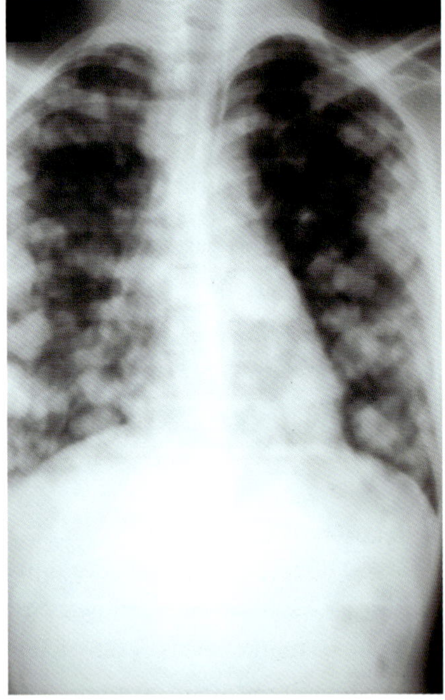

Figure 5.6 Chest radiograph film showing multiple pulmonary metastases from a testicular teratoma – these resolved following an intensive course of platinum-based chemotherapy.

In approximately 25% of men with metastatic testicular teratoma, a residual mass persists after completion of chemotherapy, and this is most commonly located in the retroperitoneum. In such patients, long-term survival of over 90% can be achieved if all residual masses are excised completely. Retroperitoneal lymph node dissection can be performed to remove residual masses through a midline abdominal incision, though a thoraco-abdominal extraperitoneal approach may be preferable (Figure 5.7). This latter approach allows synchronous excision of disease within the lung or thoracic lymph nodes and retroperitoneal nodes without breaching the peritoneal cavity, thus avoiding paralytic ileus. It is also possible to remove involved cervical lymph nodes during the same operation. Preservation of the sympathetic nerve fibres, particularly the hypogastric nerve plexus just distal to the bifurcation of the aorta, during RPLND should prevent disturbance of ejaculation.

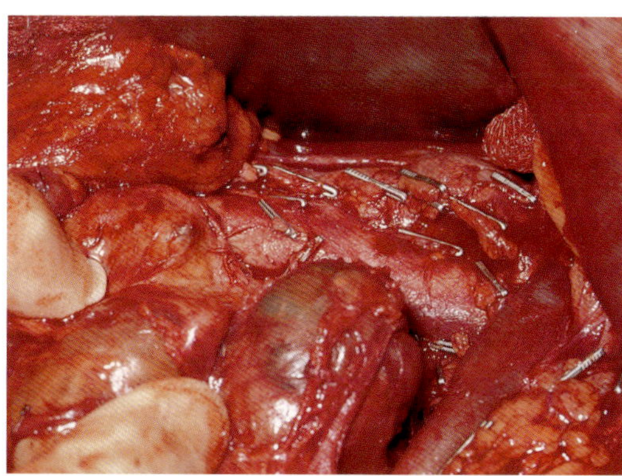

Figure 5.7 Operative view during a left-sided post-chemotherapy thoraco-abdominal retroperitoneal lymph node dissection for metastatic testicular teratoma. The mass of nodes is shown in the foreground with the abdominal aorta in the background.

Prognosis

The prognosis for stages I–II testicular cancer is excellent, with 5-year survival rates of over 95%. In more advanced tumours that are chemosensitive, the 5-year survival rate approaches 90%. The worst prognostic factors are the presence of liver and brain metastases.

CHAPTER 6

Diseases of the scrotal skin

Diseases of the scrotal skin are relatively common and can be subclassified as:

- congenital
- infectious
- benign
- malignant.

As with some diseases of the penis, many patients are reluctant to seek medical attention for such disorders until they have progressed to a dramatically extreme state.

Congenital conditions

The scrotum may be congenitally abnormal in a variety of different ways. In a few cases it may be unilaterally atrophic, be ectopic within the groin, engulf the penis, or be webbed in its attachment to the penis. Such anomalies are usually amenable to surgical reconstruction. Congenital haemangiomas are quite common, particularly the strawberry haemangioma, which often undergoes spontaneous involution. If one persists, it can be treated by neodymium:YAG laser.

Infectious diseases

The most common infectious disease that affects the scrotal skin is the fungal infection tinea cruris. The characteristic itchy, raised red patches are most often found within the skin creases of the groin, but they often spread to involve the skin of the scrotum. This condition is particularly common in men living in a hot climate and in those with poor personal hygiene. The treatment is local application of antifungal cream.

Another infectious disease of the scrotum is staphylococcal folliculitis, which can progress to form abscesses. Early stages of this condition are best treated with antibiotics (particularly flucloxacillin), but if discrete abscesses develop surgical drainage may be indicated. Sexually transmitted diseases, such as syphilis (Figure 6.1), chancroid, lymphogranuloma venereum and granuloma inguinale, may present as ulcerative skin lesions of the scrotal

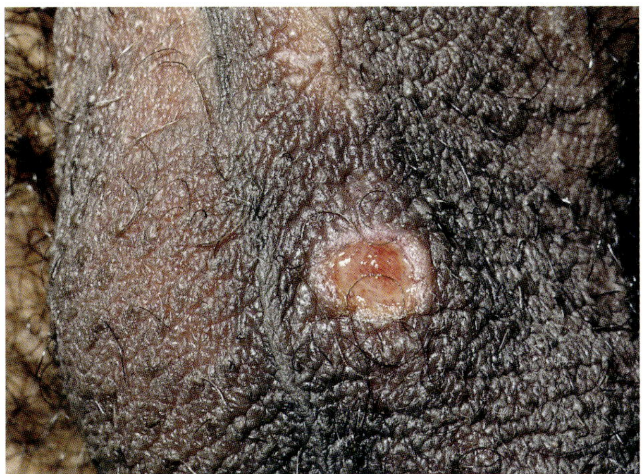

Figure 6.1 Scrotal skin ulceration due to syphilis.

skin. In tropical countries, filarial infection of the scrotal skin can lead to elephantiasis, with gross enlargement of the scrotum.

Fournier's gangrene. The most serious and potentially fatal infectious disease of the scrotal skin is Fournier's gangrene, a condition similar to necrotizing fasciitis that affects other parts of the body. This infection most often occurs in elderly diabetic men with poor personal hygiene, and alcoholics. It is often caused by a synergistic infection with Gram-negative rods and Gram-positive cocci. In the early stages of Fournier's gangrene, a small red patch appears on the scrotum, perineum or perianal area. This may rapidly progress to necrotic

Figure 6.2 Fournier's gangrene of the scrotum showing a characteristic necrotic centre with surrounding erythema.

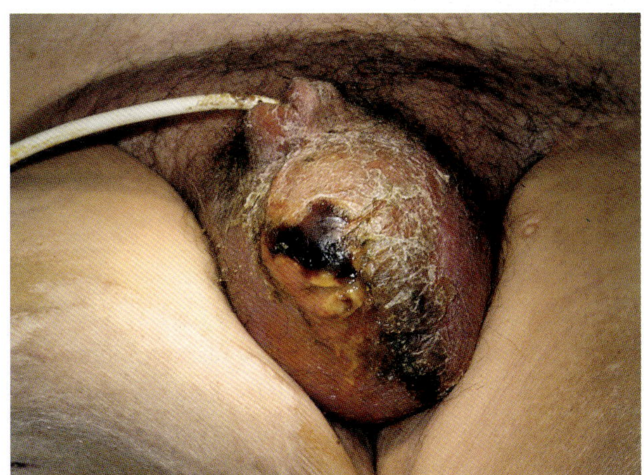

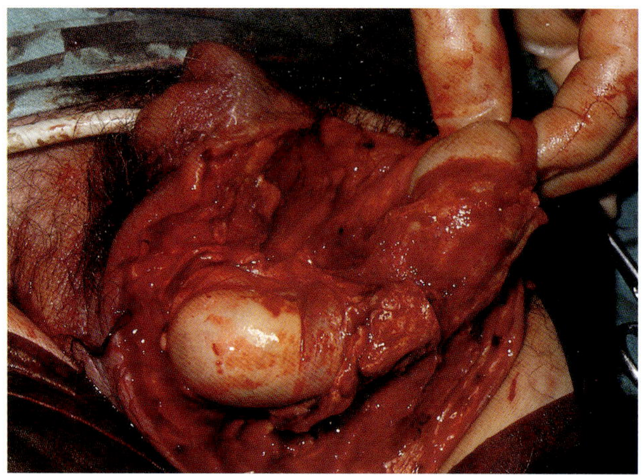

Figure 6.3 Debridement of the scrotal skin in Fournier's gangrene. The testes are apparent in the centre of the picture.

black skin with a grey colour to the surrounding skin and subcutaneous gas formation (Figure 6.2). Fifty per cent of patients presenting with Fournier's gangrene have perirectal pathology as the cause of their disease.

Management. This disease is a genuine surgical emergency, requiring prompt aggressive debridement of the scrotal skin (Figure 6.3), and sometimes also removal of involved skin and subcutaneous skin of the lower abdominal wall and inner thigh. Failure to adequately excise the tissue or delay in treatment can be fatal. Broad-spectrum antibiotics, including agents that treat Gram-positive, Gram-negative and anaerobic bacteria, are an important adjunct in the treatment of this condition. It is sometimes necessary to leave the testes floating freely in the course of debridement of the scrotum but, providing adequate debridement has been achieved, granulation of the scrotal skin will rapidly occur with dressing changes (Figure 6.4). This process can be speeded up by the addition of a split-skin graft to the scrotum.

Benign conditions of the scrotal skin

A variety of skin diseases may involve the scrotum. Perhaps the most common disorder of the scrotal skin is psoriasis, which manifests itself as raised red plaques with desquamating keratin on its surface. The treatment is the same as for psoriasis involving other areas of the body, though some prudence should be exercised in suggesting exposure of the region to sunshine! Another generalized skin condition that may involve the scrotum

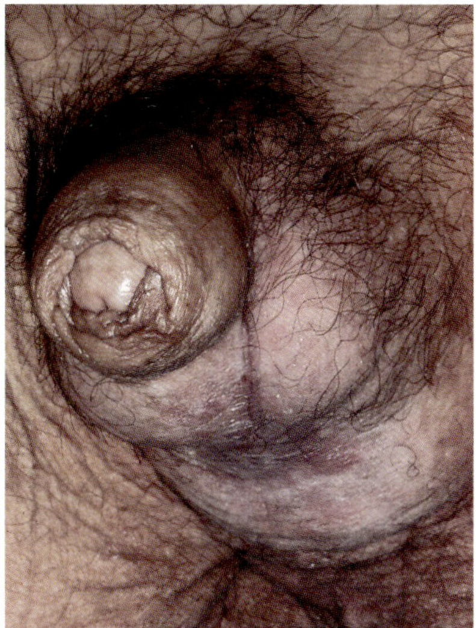

Figure 6.4 Two months following surgical debridement for Fournier's gangrene, the patient's scrotum has completely healed without further surgical intervention.

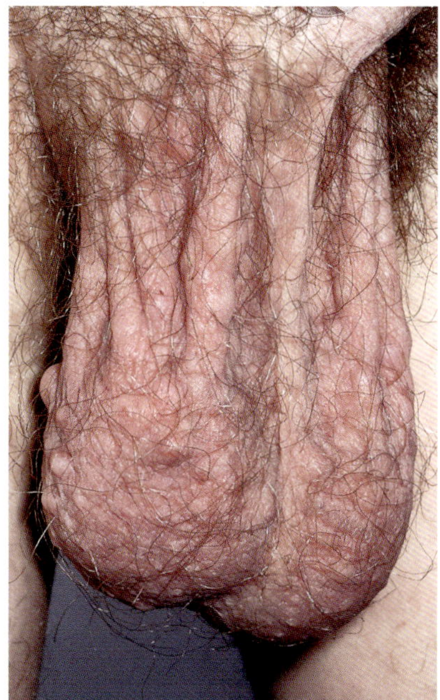

Figure 6.5 Sebaceous cysts of the scrotum.

is lichen planus, which presents as mauve-coloured raised itchy plaques of skin. Local treatment with topical steroid creams should help to relieve the condition.

The sebaceous glands of the scrotal skin are prone to develop problems in the same fashion as other areas of skin. Retention of skin secretions within glands can lead to sebaceous cysts (Figure 6.5), which run the risk of becoming infected. A rare condition of the scrotum in which sebaceous glands accumulate secretions that become calcified is sometimes referred to as scrotal calcinosis. The treatment of sebaceous cysts and scrotal calcinosis is surgical excision of each individual lesion, though conservative management is an option.

Malignant diseases of the scrotal skin

Cancer of the scrotal skin (Figure 6.6) is fortunately now a rare disease. The classic description by Percival Pott of squamous cell carcinoma of the scrotum is renowned, because this was the first malignancy to be recognized as an occupational disease, having originally been described in chimney sweeps. Repeated exposure of the scrotal skin to soot particles is thought to be the carcinogenic factor in this disease.

Management of the condition is by surgical excision of the primary tumour. Careful surveillance of the inguinal lymph nodes is important to ensure that metastatic disease does not occur. If metastases develop within the inguinal lymph nodes, inguinal lymphadenectomy is indicated and some form of adjuvant chemotherapy is advisable.

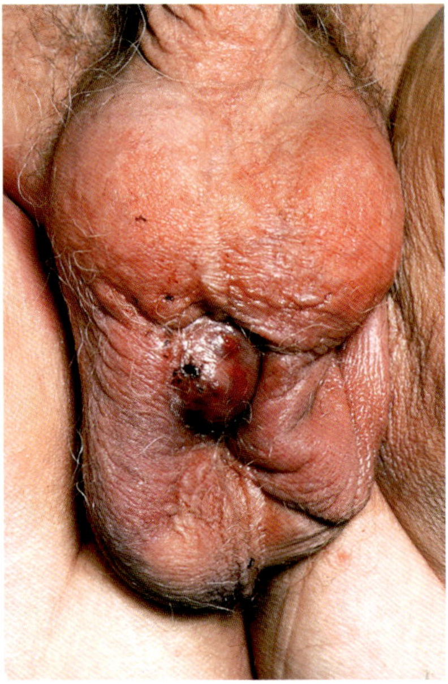

Figure 6.6 Squamous cell carcinoma arising from the scrotal skin.

Direct invasion from a primary testicular cancer is a rare but important cause of malignant ulceration of the scrotal skin. This is a very rare *de novo* finding and is more likely to occur following injudicious exploration of a testicular tumour via a scrotal incision.

Management. In these circumstances the treatment of choice is inguinal orchidectomy, followed by platinum-based chemotherapy. It is seldom necessary to excise large segments of the scrotal skin.

CHAPTER 7

Male infertility

The testes, vulnerable to systemic and environmental insult, play a vital role in a man's ability to father a child. Understanding this role is an important part of the complex process of evaluating and treating the growing number, of men seeking treatment for male infertility. The number of couples affected by infertility is currently estimated to be 15% of all couples attempting to have children. The difficulties are attributable to a significant male factor alone in 30% of couples and to a combination of male and female factors in an additional 20%. Therefore, in 50% of all infertile couples, an abnormal male factor contributes to reproductive failure.

The family practitioner is often the first healthcare professional the patient seeks, and consequently is responsible for the absolutely critical initial evaluation of the subfertile male. This evaluation involves a thorough history and physical examination and laboratory tests, including at least a semen analysis and hormonal evaluation. It may eventually be appropriate to refer the couple to an infertility specialist.

History

The information that should be sought on initial history-taking is summarized in Table 7.1 and briefly described here.

Reproductive history. In the past, fertility evaluations were delayed until a couple had been unable to achieve a pregnancy during 1 year of unprotected intercourse. It is the current philosophy that an evaluation may begin whenever a couple expresses concern, and both the man and the woman can be investigated simultaneously in an efficient, cost-effective and timely fashion. Difficulties achieving pregnancies with either past or present partners, the age of the male partner when any pregnancy occurred, and any previous evaluations or treatments should be noted.

Childhood illnesses and disorders. Several of these may predispose to infertility in men.

Delayed or incomplete puberty may reveal an endocrinological aetiology,

TABLE 7.1

Extensive history-taking is necessary in infertile men to identify any possible causative factors

Male reproductive history

- Duration of unprotected intercourse
- Previous pregnancies
- Previous infertility evaluations

Female reproductive history

- Age
- Gravida/para
- Physician's name
- Ovulation with technique to assess
- Current status of female infertility evaluation

Family history

- Cystic fibrosis
- Androgen receptor deficiency
- Hypogonadism

Endocrine history

- Headaches, visual disturbances, anosmia
- Excessive growth of hands, feet, jaw
- Retardation of hair growth (facial, body)
- Breast changes
- Vasomotor symptoms

Personal history

- Developmental
  - puberty (normal/delayed/precocious)
  - history of undescended testes
  - history of gynaecomastia
- Surgical
  - pelvic surgery (Y-V plasty to bladder neck, transurethral surgery)
  - inguinal surgery (herniorrhaphy, orchidopexy)
- Gonadotrophins
  - occupational
  - thermal exposure (saunas, hot tubs, briefs)
  - radiation exposure (work, diagnostic, therapeutic)
  - chemical exposure (work, therapeutic)
  - smoking (marijuana, cigarettes)
  - alcohol
- Sexual history
  - potency/libido
  - coital technique
  - timing and frequency of intercourse
  - use of lubricants
- Medication
  - maternal (oestrogens)
  - personal use
  - steroids

such as Klinefelter's syndrome or idiopathic hypogonadism. Similarly, gynaecomastia may also suggest an underlying endocrine problem.

Cryptorchidism, both unilateral and bilateral, is often associated with oligospermia. Although about 30% of men with unilateral cryptorchidism and 50% of men with bilateral cryptorchidism have sperm densities below 20 million/ml, about 80% of the former are fertile. In contrast, the fertility rate is only 50% for couples in whom the man has a history of bilateral cryptorchidism. Testes remaining undescended until after puberty do not function well, and fertility rates are not improved by postpubertal orchidopexy.

Testicular trauma or torsion. About 30–40% of men with a history of unilateral testicular torsion have an abnormal semen analysis for reasons that remain unclear. A breakdown in the blood–testis barrier may be the cause, or the testis susceptible to torsion may have had a pre-existing spermatogenic defect, as impaired spermatogenesis in the contralateral testis is common. When trauma or torsion occurs after puberty, the resultant infertility may be immunologically mediated.

Bilateral mumps orchitis, when experienced prepubertally, seems to have no effect, but mumps orchitis experienced postpubertally is associated with severe testicular damage in 10% of patients.

Previous surgery. History of bladder, pelvic or retroperitoneal surgery may suggest the possibility of ejaculatory dysfunction, with associated incomplete or retrograde ejaculation. History of a herniorrhaphy suggests the possibility of an iatrogenic vasal injury.

Environmental factors. Exposure to certain medications, drugs or environmental toxins may affect testicular function (Table 7.2). The elevated testicular temperature associated with cryptorchidism and scrotal varicoceles may explain the impaired spermatogenesis in these disorders. Men are encouraged to avoid saunas and hot baths. Any patient who has been treated with radiation or chemotherapy for testicular or other cancer is at risk of impaired spermatogenesis. Patients with testicular cancer are particularly affected.

Sexual habits. The optimal timing for intercourse is once every 48 hours during the time when ovulation is most likely, usually at the woman's

TABLE 7.2

A wide variety of medications, toxins and drugs have been associated with male infertility, and evidence of their use should be sought in the initial history-taking

Medications	Toxins
• Androgenic steroids	• Agent Orange
• Antihypertensives	• Anaesthetic gases
• Cancer chemotherapy	• Benzene
• H_2 blockers	• Dibromochloropropane (DBCP)
• Ketoconazole	• Lead
• Nitrofurantoin	• Manganese
• Spironolactone	
• Sulphasalazine	**Other drugs**
• Colchicine	• Alcohol
• Allopurinol	• Heroin
• Tetracycline	• Marijuana
• Erythromycin	• Methadone
• Gentamicin	• Tobacco
• Cyclosporin	

mid-cycle. Couples must be cautioned to use lubricants only if necessary, and then only in limited amounts. Spermatotoxic lubricants, such as K-Y Jelly, Lubifax, Surgilube, Keri Lotion, and even saliva, can impair sperm motility. Other lubricants, such as raw egg-white, vegetable oil, safflower oil, peanut oil and petroleum jelly, do not impair *in-vivo* motility.

Acquired or congenital conditions. Any inflammatory process that involves the lower urinary tract may lead to scarring of the ductal system (e.g. ejaculatory duct stenosis or obstruction), which may affect fertility. Any generalized febrile episode may transiently impair spermatogenesis. Non-motile sperm secondary to an ultrastructural defect in the sperm tail (immotile cilia syndrome) may cause infertility in men with recurrent respiratory infections (Kartagener's syndrome or Young's syndrome). Genes for cystic fibrosis are carried unknowingly by a number of men who may also have congenital absence of the vasa and seminal vesicles and, consequently, a low ejaculate volume and azoospermia. Diabetes mellitus or multiple sclerosis can impair potency as well as ejaculation.

Physical examination

The initial physical examination may reveal critical information on the aetiology of the man's infertility. Special care should be taken to note any evidence of hypogonadism or a hypothalamic or pituitary tumour. Gynaecomastia may indicate primary testicular failure or a secondary hypothalamic–pituitary axis abnormality.

Because the seminiferous tubules account for 85% of the testicular volume, a careful examination of the testicles may help to identify the cause of the infertility as testicular or post-testicular (obstructive). The size of the testes can be easily measured using a ruler, caliper or orchidometer. If testicular insult has occurred before puberty, the testicles will probably be small and firm, whereas postpubertal damage usually leaves the testicles small and soft.

The prostate should be carefully assessed: it is often small in men with androgen deficiency, and tender and boggy with prostatitis. The penis should be examined for hypospadias, abnormal curvature or phimosis, which may interfere with the proper deposition of sperm deep within the vagina. The epididymis should be palpated for irregularities that may indicate infection or obstruction, and the presence of the vas confirmed by palpation. About 2% of infertile men have congenital absence of the vasa and seminal vesicles; these men may also be carriers for cystic fibrosis genes and should undergo genetic evaluation. The testicular cords should be carefully palpated for the presence of a varicocele, as described on page 30.

When any abnormalities are noted on genital examination, prompt referral to the urologist is indicated for further non-invasive examinations, including ultrasonography, or possible surgical consideration.

A full physical examination should be performed to rule out any chronic or unsuspected systemic diseases that may impair testicular function.

Laboratory analysis

Preliminary analysis should include two properly collected semen samples and evaluation of serum FSH levels. The importance of proper specimen collection, and analysis by a laboratory that has demonstrated quality control in evaluating semen samples and regularly performs such analyses cannot be overemphasized. Abnormalities in semen samples (Table 7.3) or elevated FSH levels suggest intrinsic testicular failure with a compensatory increase in FSH production by the pituitary gland. Prompt urological referral is appropriate in such cases.

Semen analysis. Semen should be collected for analysis after 48–72 hours of abstinence from sexual intercourse, kept at body temperature and analysed within 1 hour. A minimum of two samples should be obtained after similar periods of sexual abstinence.

The semen is assessed for volume, sperm density, sperm motility, forward progression, sperm morphology and the presence of leucocytes that might indicate infection or inflammation (Table 7.3). According to the new WHO criteria, normal semen samples contain at least 30% morphologically normal sperm. Increased numbers of abnormally shaped sperm are

TABLE 7.3

Normal values of semen variables. These values represent a standard of adequacy and do not indicate that the sperm are actually able to fertilize *in vivo*

Volume	2.0 ml or more
pH	7.2–8.0
Sperm concentration	20 million/ml or more
Total sperm count	40 million or more (per ejaculate)
Motility	50% or more with forward progression, or 25% or more with rapid progression
Morphology	30% or more with normal forms
Vitality	75% or more live
White blood cells	Less than 1 million
Immunobead	Less than 20% bound

From WHO Laboratory Manual for the Examination of Human Semen and Sperm–Cervical Mucus Interaction. 3rd ed. Cambridge: University Press, 1992:44.

indicative of testicular stress (e.g. varicocele, poor sperm production or environmental toxins). It should be remembered that the laboratory analysis does not predict fertility, and that pregnancy is the only irrefutable proof of the sperm's capability to fertilize.

Measurement of anti-sperm antibodies, a sperm–cervical mucus interaction test, determination of strict sperm morphology, and the sperm penetration test are more complex assays, and are generally undertaken by a specialist in male reproductive disorders if required.

Hormonal evaluation. The prevalence of primary endocrine defects in infertile men is less than 3%, and they almost never occur in men whose sperm concentration is greater than 5×10^6/ml. Specific hormonal treatment is often successful when hormone production is deficient, though 1 year of treatment may be required to reach optimal sperm production. A hormone evaluation should therefore be performed when the sperm concentration is low or when an endocrinopathy is suspected clinically. The clinical diagnoses that can be correlated with hormonal status are shown in Table 7.4.

A markedly elevated serum FSH is usually associated with azoospermia or severe oligospermia and usually indicates primary testicular failure. A very low or non-detectable FSH level indicates hypogonadotrophic hypogonadism, which is suggested clinically by undermasculinization. Concomitantly decreased levels of serum testosterone and LH confirm the

TABLE 7.4

Although only 3% of infertile men have a primary endocrine defect, in these men the hormonal status can be correlated to the clinical diagnosis

Clinical status	FSH (mIU/ml)	LH (mIU/ml)	Testosterone (ng/100 ml)
Normal men	Normal	Normal	Normal
Germinal aplasia	Elevated	Normal	Normal or decreased
Testicular failure	Elevated	Elevated	Normal or decreased
Hypogonadotrophic hypogonadism	Decreased	Decreased	Decreased
Hypergonadotrophic hypogonadism	Elevated	Elevated	Low–normal or decreased

diagnosis. Because hyperprolactinaemia has also been reported to cause oligospermia, serum prolactin should be measured when a patient has a low serum testosterone level without an associated increase in LH, as well as symptoms of decreased libido, decreased ejaculate volume and evidence of galactorrhoea.

Specialist referral

Once a thorough history and physical examination have been completed and the appropriate laboratory tests have been performed, referral to a urology specialist in the field of male reproductive medicine and surgery can be considered. With proper evaluation and appropriate referral, male factor problems are increasingly treated with success, and previously infertile couples are able to enjoy the rewards of parenthood.

Management

Management of severe male factor infertility has been revolutionized by the introduction of intracytoplasmic sperm injection (ICSI) (Figure 7.1). Men with conditions previously considered untreatable, such as congenital bilateral absence of the vas deferens or severe oligospermia, are now potentially able to initiate a pregnancy with ICSI. Although the first success using this technique was reported as recently as 1992, ICSI is now being

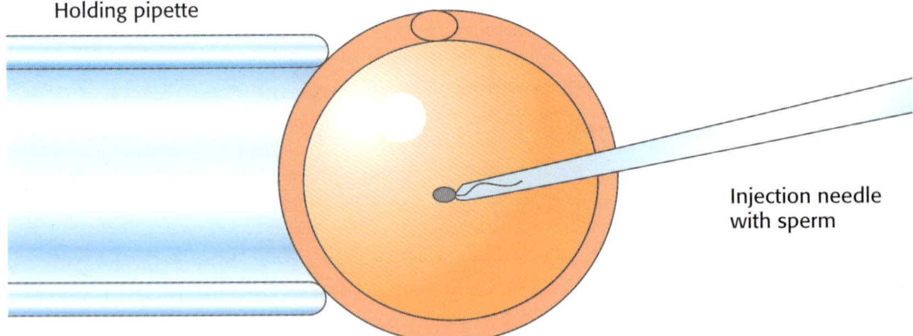

Figure 7.1 During intracytoplasmic sperm injection (ICSI), a single sperm is injected into a processed egg held on a special pipette. This technique can be used to initiate a pregnancy with sperm from men whose infertility was previously considered to be untreatable.

performed by most major *in-vitro* fertilization (IVF) centres in the world.

Sperm for ICSI may be obtained from the ejaculate, the epididymis or even the testis itself. The best ICSI fertilization rates are reported when ejaculated sperm is used, and this is the source of choice. Even in the presence of marked defects in sperm density, motility and/or morphology, normal fertilization is achievable in up to 70% of injected oocytes.

Microscopic epididymal sperm aspiration (**MESA**) can be used to obtain sperm in men with surgically untreatable obstructive azoospermia or congenital bilateral absence of the vas deferens. Because of typically normal spermatogenesis, numerous sperm are obtained with MESA. The outcome of MESA in combination with ICSI is significantly better in terms of fertilization, clinical pregnancy and ongoing pregnancy/delivery rates, than in combination with conventional IVF. Up to 60% of men with congenital bilateral absence of the vas deferens carry a cystic fibrosis gene, and testing both partners is, therefore, critical. If both partners are carriers, pre-implantation embryo blastomere biopsy must be considered. Cryopreservation of sperm from azoospermic men undergoing MESA is strongly recommended as thawed spermatozoa give a high success rate.

Percutaneous epididymal sperm aspiration (**PESA**) is simple and highly successful. Adequate numbers of spermatozoa can be obtained from nearly 90% of patients, with a subsequent mean fertilization rate of about 33%. Caveats regarding PESA include the blind nature of the procedure with potential damage to the delicate epididymal tubules, thereby limiting future epididymal sperm recovery. The recovery of adequate numbers of sperm for cryopreservation, to enable future ICSI attempts, is also severely limited.

Testicular sperm extraction (**TESE**) combined with ICSI has been used for azoospermic men when no sperm can be recovered from the epididymis. In patients with complete absence of the epididymis or massive scarring from previous surgery, an open biopsy of the testis is usually performed. After the testis tissue is minced in a sperm preparation medium, sperm are selected by micropipette under microscopic guidance. Needle aspiration of the testis is also possible (TESA). The fertilization and pregnancy rates with TESE are generally slightly lower than with ejaculated or epididymal sperm.

Possible birth defects. There are no convincing data to support concerns about an increased risk of birth defects with ICSI. In addition, concerns regarding sex predilection have not been confirmed. Careful investigation of the male ICSI offspring will determine whether the abnormalities present in the father will be transmitted to the male offspring with resultant infertility. Screening is currently in progress for Y chromosome defects, such as absence of the *DAZ* gene in the *AZF* region, which may be responsible for certain types of male factor infertility.

CHAPTER 8

Future trends

Testicular cancer

Testicular cancer remains the most common malignancy in young men, and its incidence is increasing. There is a strong body of evidence that early detection of these tumours is advantageous both in terms of the long-term prognosis and the avoidance of chemotherapy with its side-effects. Screening programmes have been started in some Scandinavian countries, but these have not yet been proven to be of clinical benefit. Testicular self-examination is now being strongly advocated in many countries. An increase in public awareness of testicular cancer through advertising programmes may well prove to be effective in detecting this disease at an earlier stage in its natural history.

The role of RPLND in stages I and II testicular teratoma remains controversial. Some centres advocate surveillance for stage I tumours, while others perform RPLND even though the nodes are clear of tumour in up to 70% of cases. A similar dilemma exists for stage II testicular cancer; the relative merits of immediate RPLND followed by chemotherapy in the case of relapse, or chemotherapy followed by RPLND in the event of relapse remain controversial. The cure rate for metastatic testicular cancer is now so high that it is perhaps more pertinent to compare the morbidity of RPLND with that of chemotherapy in reaching clinical decisions in the clinical management of these young men. However, long-term prospective randomized clinical trials focusing on both cure rates and the morbidity of RPLND and contemporary chemotherapy regimens will hopefully answer some of these questions.

Following chemotherapy for stage II–IV testicular cancer, most urologists advocate RPLND for residual tumour masses greater than 2 cm in diameter. However, in 15–50% of cases, the resected tissue appears to be completely necrotic and it could be argued that, in such circumstances, surgery is unnecessary. We are currently unable to differentiate necrotic tissue from differentiated teratoma and actively malignant tissue using most imaging techniques, although elevated tumour markers do suggest the presence of persistent malignant activity. Recent research into newer imaging techniques such as PET scanning and radioimmunoscintigraphy offers some hope in identifying the presence and location of active malignancy in these patients. Such techniques may, in the future, permit more precise selection for surgical intervention in men with active malignancy.

Infective conditions

Our understanding of the aetiology, pathogenesis and treatment of epididymo-orchitides is constantly improving. Effective screening for organisms such as *Chlamydia* and those responsible for other sexually transmitted diseases should significantly reduce the incidence of infection. Improvements in antibiotic therapy – particularly the quinolones – leading to better tissue penetration and longer half-lives will improve the efficacy and reduce the dosage frequency of such drugs.

Infertility

Improvements in IVF techniques and the development of single gamete micromanipulation (i.e. intracytoplasmic sperm injection/ICSI) have led to novel treatments for men with otherwise untreatable testicular failure or genital tract obstruction. These new techniques allow injection of a single sperm into an oocyte that has been retrieved through the process of ovarian hyperstimulation.

Although sperm for IVF may be obtained from either ejaculated, epididymal or testicular 'reservoirs', it is use of sperm from the last of these (i.e. via testicular sperm extraction/TESE) that has allowed men with the most significant defects of sperm production to father their own biological children.

Current data indicate that the incidence of gross congenital anomalies is not increased when testicular sperm are used for achieving pregnancies. However, new genetic testing procedures are being used to determine whether chromosomal defects might be transmitted via the ICSI technique. Furthermore, some patients who have undergone multiple TESE cycles have experienced a decrease in testosterone production due to loss of testicular volume and associated testicular devascularization. Thus, although TESE offers new hope to patients with even the most severe defects in sperm production, some important questions remain unanswered.

Interest in the testis as a source of sperm, even for otherwise azoospermic patients, has stimulated renewed scientific investigation into the aetiology of testicular failure. Two new concepts are receiving considerable attention: the role of apoptosis in impaired spermatogenesis, and the increased incidence of mitotic/meiotic failure, as demonstrated by fluorescent *in-situ* hybridization (FISH) in patients with decreased sperm maturation.

Apoptosis is an active phenomenon resulting in cell death and represents a final common pathway in response to various stimuli and forms of cell cycle regulation. Recent studies have demonstrated increased apoptotic activity in the human seminiferous epithelium that exhibits patterns such as hypospermatogenesis and maturation arrest. These findings indicate that apoptosis may play a key regulatory role in the dynamic process of human spermatogenesis.

FISH has also been used extensively to look at sperm from individuals with impaired testicular function, and to identify increased aneuploidy. Recent work, however, has quantified aneuploidy in testis biopsies themselves. Surprisingly, increased aneuploidy was found not only during meiosis, as expected, but also to an even greater extent during mitosis. This would indicate, perhaps, a potential genetic defect in checkpoint regulation of early germ cell division.

Both of these techniques – apoptosis quantitation and FISH analysis – are leading to a new understanding of the causes of male infertility and, hopefully, will provide guidance in the development of effective new therapies.

Key references

TUMOURS OF THE TESTIS

Doherty AP, Bower M, Christmas TJ. The role of tumour markers in the diagnosis and treatment of testicular germ cell tumours. *Br J Urol* 1997;79:247–52.

Donohue JP. Unsolved problems in testis cancer. *Eur Urol* 1993;23:57–9.

Donohue JP, Zachary JM, Maynard BR. Distribution of nodal metastases in nonseminomatous testis cancer. *J Urol* 1982;128:315–20.

Hendry WF, A'Hern RP, Hetherington JW, Peckham MJ, Dearnaley DP, Horwich A. Para-aortic lymphadenectomy after chemotherapy for metastatic non-seminomatous germ cell tumours: prognostic value and therapeutic benefit. *Br J Urol* 1993;71:208–13.

Moul JW, Dodge RK, Robertson JE, Paulson DF, Walther PJ. The impact of the "cisplatin era" of treatment on survival in testicular cancer. *World J Urol* 1991;9:45–50.

MALE INFERTILITY

Gilbert BR, Schlegel PN, Goldstein M. Office evaluation of the subfertile male. AUA Update Series 1994: volume 13, lesson 9, 69–76.

Howards SS. Treatment of male infertility. *N Engl J Med* 1995;332:312–17.

In't Veld P, Brandenburg H, Verhoeff A, Dhont M, Los F. Sex chromosomal abnormalities and intracytoplasmic sperm injection. *Lancet* 1995;346:773.

Lipshultz LI (guest editor). Male infertility. *Urol Clin North Am* 1994;21.

Lipshultz LI, Howards SS, Buch JP. Male infertility. In: Gillenwater JY, Grayhack JT, Howards SS, Duckett JW, eds. *Adult and Pediatric Urology*. 2nd ed. St Louis: Mosby Year Book, 1991:1425–78.

McClure RD. Male infertility. In: Tanagho EA, McAnich JW, eds. *Smith's General Urology*. London: Prentice Hall International, 1995:739–71.

Nagy ZP, Liu J, Cecile J, Silber S, Devroey P, Van Steirteghem A. Using ejaculated, fresh, and frozen-thawed epididymal and testicular spermatozoa gives rise to comparable results after intracytoplasmic sperm injection. *Fertil Steril* 1995;63: 808–15.

Nagy ZP, Verheyen G, Liu J *et al.* Results of 55 intracytoplasmic sperm injection cycles in the treatment of male immunological infertility. *Hum Reprod* 1995;10:1775–80.

Schlegel PN, Palermo GD, Alikani M *et al.* Micropuncture retrieval of epididymal sperm with in vitro fertilization: importance of in vitro micromanipulation techniques. *Urology* 1995;46:238–41.

Sigman M, Howards SS. Male infertility. In: Walsh PC, Retik AB, Stamey TA, Vaughn DA Jr, eds. *Campbell's Urology*. Philadelphia: WB Saunders, 1992:659–705.

Silber SJ, Van Steirteghem AC, Liu J, Nagy Z, Tournaye H, Devroey P. High fertilization and pregnancy rate after intracytoplasmic sperm injection with spermatozoa obtained from testicle biopsy. *Hum Reprod* 1995;10:148–52.

Index

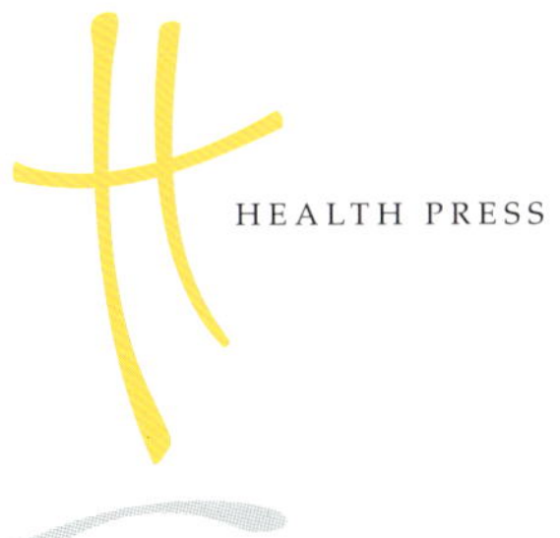

Also available

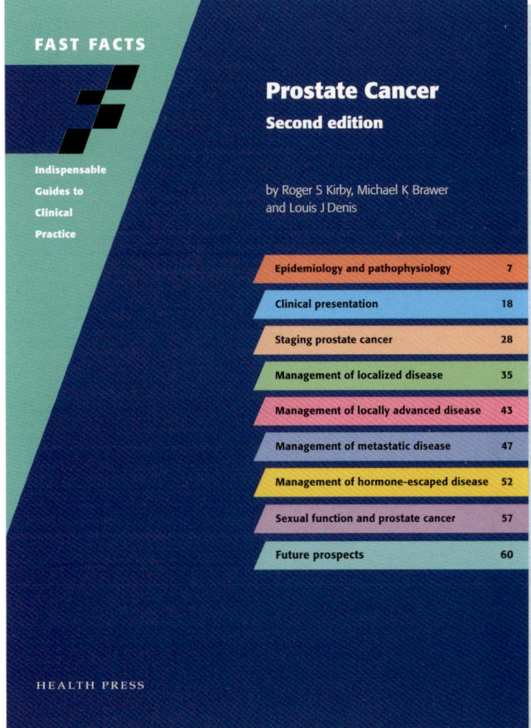

- Epidemiology and pathophysiology
- Clinical presentation
- Staging prostate cancer
- Management of localized disease
- Management of locally advanced disease
- Management of metastatic disease
- Management of hormone-escaped disease
- Sexual function and prostate cancer
- Future prospects

FAST FACTS

Prostate Cancer Second edition

by Roger S Kirby, Michael K Brawer and Louis J Denis

Prostate cancer is now a major concern for our ageing male populations. Yet rapid scientific advances leave the family practitioner faced with new and often controversial ideas. So what are the essential facts needed for the diagnosis and management of this insidious disease? Three leading urologists from the UK, USA and Belgium present a clear and concise consensus in this immensely practical book.

ISBN: 1-899541-42-X; Page extent: 68 pages; First published: 1998; UK £10.95 each; overseas £11.95 or US $19.95 each.

Also available

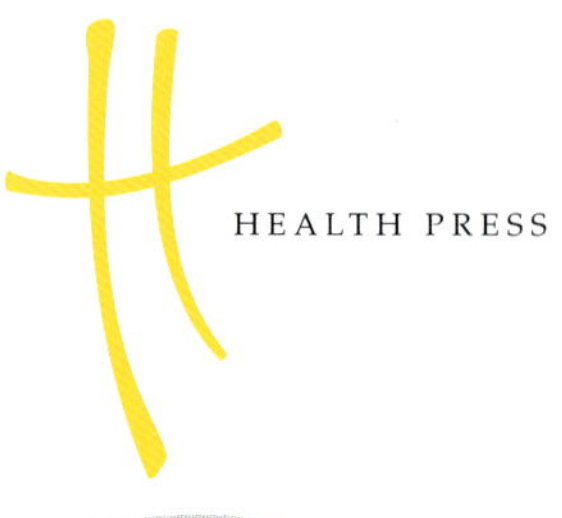

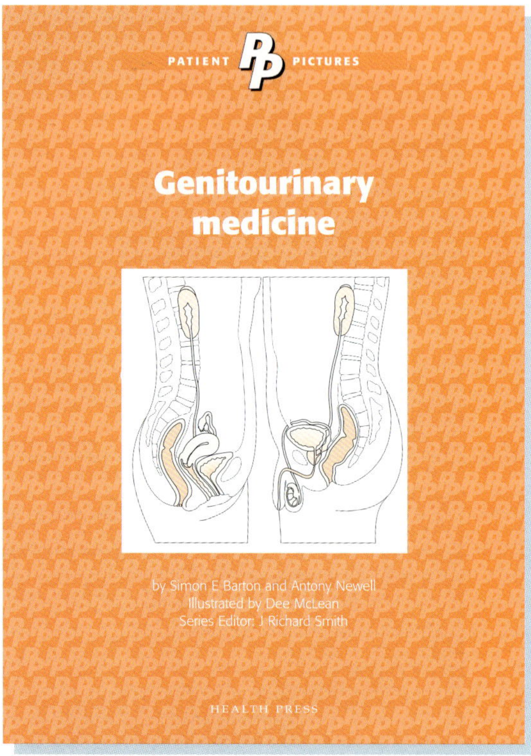

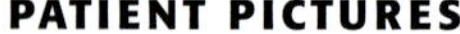

PATIENT PICTURES

Genitourinary medicine

by Simon E Barton and Antony Newell

- The male genitourinary tract
- The female genitourinary tract
- First clinic visit
- Tests

Men

- Urethritis
- Gonorrhoea
- Genital warts
- Genital herpes
- Epididymo-orchitis
- Perianal conditions
- Proctitis
- Prostatitis

Women

- Vaginal discharge
- Thrush
- Bacterial vaginosis
- Cervical infections
- Gonorrhoea
- *Trichomonas vaginalis*
- *Chlamydia trachomatis*
- Genital warts
- Genital herpes
- Perianal conditions
- Pelvic inflammatory disease (PID)
- Cystitis

General

- Syphilis
- Hepatitis B
- HIV infection
- Contact tracing and follow-up

Many people feel anxious about visiting a genitourinary medicine clinic, often because they feel embarrassed or worried. As a result, it can be very difficult to remember or absorb everything that is said.

In order for treatment to be effective, it is vital that a patient understands the nature of the infection, how it was contracted, the treatment prescribed and the importance of contacting sexual partners. This book is intended for healthcare professionals to use with their patients to help achieve this goal.

ISBN 1-899541-32-2; Page extent: 62 pages; First published: 1999; UK £10.95 each; overseas £11.95 or US $19.95 each.

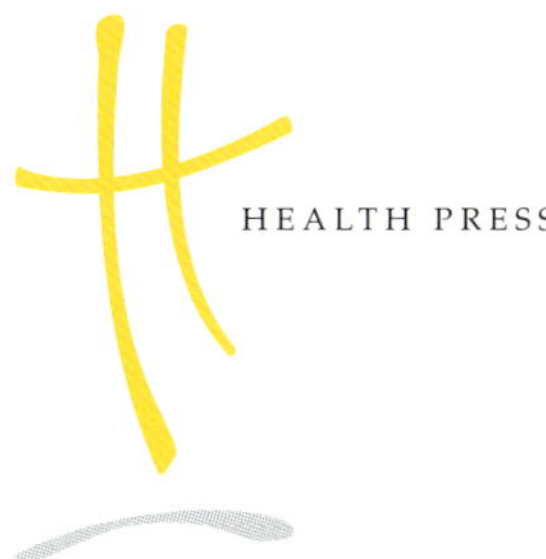

Also available

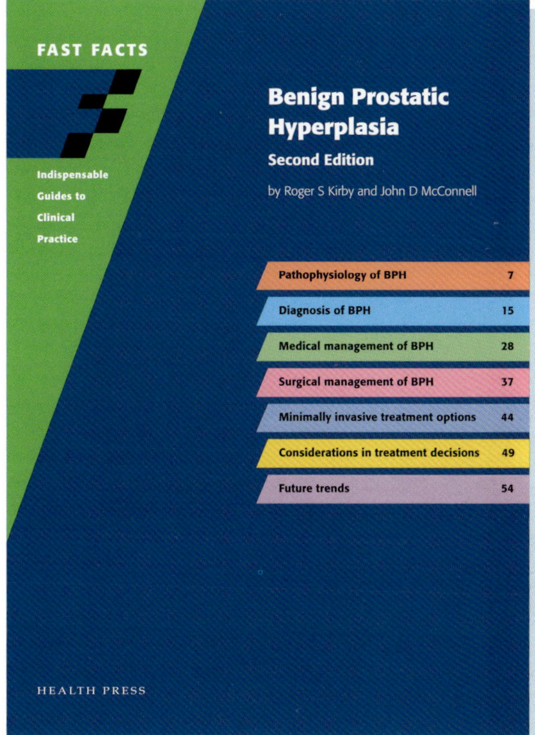

- Pathophysiology of BPH
- Diagnosis of BPH
- Medical management of BPH
- Surgical management of BPH
- Minimally invasive treatment options
- Considerations in treatment decisions
- Future trends

FAST FACTS

Benign Prostatic Hyperplasia **Second edition**

by Roger S Kirby and John D McConnell

Written with the family physician and specialist nurse in mind, this book reviews the most appropriate treatment options for this increasingly prevalent disease.

ISBN: 1-899541-81-0; Page extent: 64 pages; First published: 1997; UK £10.95 each; overseas £11.95 or US $19.95 each.

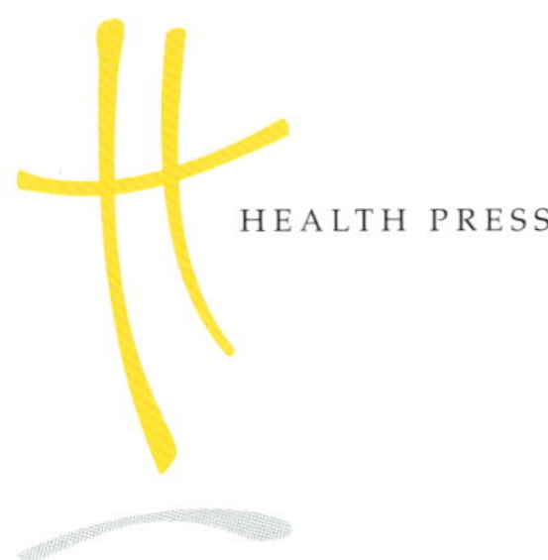

Also available

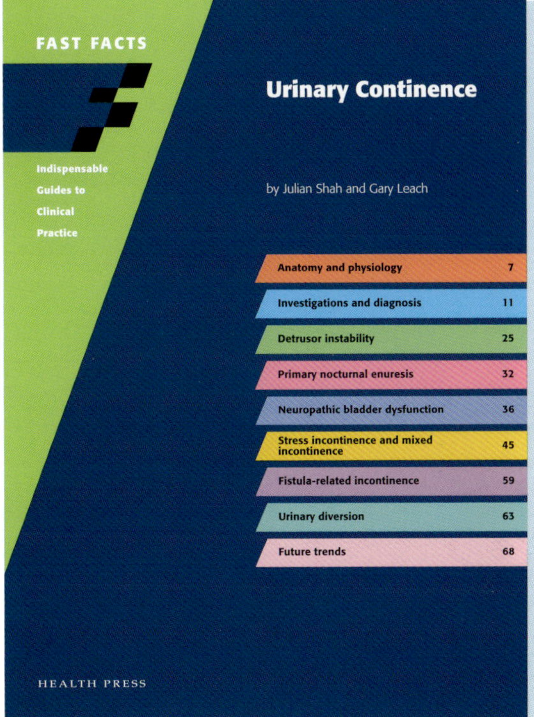

- Anatomy and physiology
- Investigations and diagnosis
- Detrusor instability
- Primary nocturnal enuresis
- Neuropathic bladder dysfunction
- Stress incontinence and mixed incontinence
- Fistula-related incontinence
- Urinary diversion
- Future trends

FAST FACTS

Urinary Continence

by Julian Shah and Gary Leach

Urinary incontinence is a source of great distress to sufferers and their relatives. But nowadays, most patients can be diagnosed and treated with minimal investigation. Written for family physicians, hospital doctors and specialist nurses, *Fast Facts – Urinary Continence* outlines the current approach to management of this most embarrassing of problems.

ISBN: 1-899541-65-9; Page extent: 76 pages; First published: 1998; UK £10.95 each; overseas £11.95 or US $19.95 each.